EASY EXERCISES FOR CORE FITNESS

The Stay Fit Series

A Special Report published
by the editors of *Healthy Years*
in conjunction with
The David Geffen School of Medicine at UCLA
Division of Geriatrics

Easy Exercises for Core Fitness

Consulting Editor: Ellen G. Wilson, PT, Director of Therapy Services, UCLA Health

Author: Jim Brown, PhD, Executive Editor, Steadman Philippon Research Institute
Group Directors, Belvoir Media Group: Diane Muhlfeld, Jay Roland
Creative Director, Belvoir Media Group: Judi Crouse
Belvoir Editor: Matthew Solan
Illustrators: Alayna Paquette, Marty Bee, Thinkstock

Publisher, Belvoir Media Group: Timothy H. Cole

ISBN 978-1-879620-99-5

To order additional copies of this report or for customer service questions, please call 877-300-0253, or write to
Health Special Reports, 535 Connecticut Avenue, Norwalk, CT 06854.

NEW FINDINGS

- Trunk muscle strength is associated with improved balance, daily functions, and prevention of falls (Page 8, Box 1-1).

- Moderate-intensity exercise improves mobility (Page 11, Box 1-4).

- Light daily physical activity reduces disability (Page 11, Box 1-5).

- Resistance training offsets the loss of muscle mass associated with aging (Page 12, Box 1-6).

- Core strength improves spinal and functional mobility (Page 12, Box 1-7).

- Exercise programs reduce the risk of falls and injuries caused by falls (Page 13, Box 1-8).

- Foam rollers ease muscle fatigue and soreness (Page 16, Box 2-3).

- Half of exercise program participants drop out (Page 17, Box 2-4).

- Goal setting and instructor feedback help participants adhere to an exercise program (Page 17, Box 2-5).

- Chair-based exercise develops core strength (Page 21, Box 2-7).

- Core muscle strength improves balance (Page 25, Box 2-9).

- More muscle mass in older adults reduces the risk of dying prematurely (Page 32, Box 3-4).

- Low vitamin D in blood is associated with a higher risk of premature death (Page 34, Box 3-6).

Easy Exercises for
Core Fitness

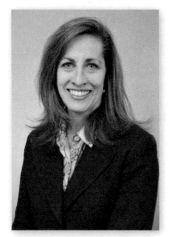

Ellen G. Wilson, PT
Director of Therapy Services
UCLA Health

A Message from the David Geffen School of Medicine at UCLA and Ellen G. Wilson, PT, Director of Therapy Services, UCLA Health

"**W**elcome to *Easy Exercises for Core Fitness* Special Report. Some of the most important muscles in the body are those in the hips, pelvis, abdomen, and trunk. Together, they are called the core, and they are involved in every aspect of our daily routines—getting up, lying down, sitting, standing, moving, maintaining balance, and enjoying a healthy lifestyle. Yet, most people take the core for granted, and few are aware of why it is so important.

The information and exercises in last year's *Easy Exercises for Balance & Mobility* Special Report have given some of you a head start. But good balance requires a strong core, and *Easy Exercises for Core Fitness* gives every reader a fresh start. It goes beyond balance and mobility, and shows you how to become stronger, more flexible, and more independent, regardless of your age or fitness level.

This edition describes and illustrates 50 exercises using inexpensive equipment many people have at home, as well as programs that will add enjoyment to your choice of physical activity—walking, jogging, swimming, tennis, golf, bowling, gardening, and others.

Illustrations, charts, tables, lists, and sample week-long workout logs will help you get started or increase your level of core fitness. 'New Findings' will update you on research that could have an immediate impact on your daily activities.

On behalf of all of us at UCLA, thanks for your interest in becoming and staying physically fit. We want this report to help you live a longer, healthier, and more productive life. Working toward core fitness is a great way to start."

Table of Contents

NEW FINDINGS 3

A PREVIEW 6

1 THE CORE CONNECTION 8

What is the core? 8

How the core affects daily activities 10

  Flexibility 10

  Strength 10

  Injuries 12

  Falls/balance 12

Signs that core muscles need work 12

  Poor posture 12

  Lower back pain 13

  Weakness 13

What's next? 13

2 GETTING READY 14

Warm up 16

Cool down 16

Sticking with the program 17

Equipment options 18

  Body weight 18

  Stability balls 18

  Free weights (dumbbells) 20

  Chair-based exercises 20

  Resistance bands 20

  Medicine balls 21

Yoga, tai chi, and Pilates 22

  Yoga 22

  Tai chi 23

  Pilates 23

Walking 24

Testing for core fitness 24

  Self-test 25

Good posture 25

It's never too late 27

What's next? 27

3 PREVENTING INJURIES 28

Strains 28

  Symptoms 29

  Treatment 29

  Prevention: 10 tips 29

Sprains 30

  Symptoms 30

  Treatment 31

  Prevention 31

Cramps 31

  Treatment 32

  Prevention 32

Muscle imbalance 32

  How do you know? 32

Longevity 33

Muscle mass loss 33

The nutrition factor 34

  Short-term: Dealing with the
    stress of exercise 34

What's next? 35

4 EASY EXERCISES 36

The directory 36

The exercises 36

What's next? 36

Easy exercises number and page directory 37

5 THE WORKBOOK 54

Strength programs 55

Flexibility programs 56

Balance programs 57

Monthly program workbook 58

Activity and sports programs 60

APPENDIX I: GLOSSARY 62

APPENDIX II: RESOURCES 64

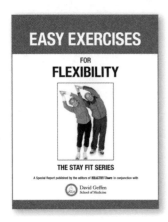

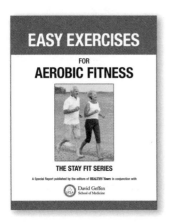

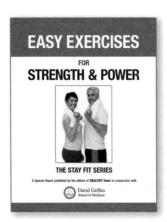

Easy Exercises for
Core Fitness

A PREVIEW

Chapter 1, *The Core Connection,* explains what the core is and why it is important to every movement you make every day, all day. The chapter also shows you where these important groups of muscles lie, how they work, and why they are essential for strength, flexibility, and balance. And, perhaps most important, this chapter will help you identify the signs of weak core muscles and get you started toward making them stronger.

▶ **Chapter 2,** *Getting Ready,* takes you through the steps to ensure success with your exercise program. What should you wear to work out? How often should you exercise? How long? How hard? What equipment will you need? You also need to test your current core fitness and learn how to maintain good standing and sitting posture to ensure you can safely practice many of the core muscle movements.

▶ **Chapter 3,** *Preventing Injuries.* People who exercise occasionally suffer an injury along the way. Avoid pulled muscles, sprains, and cramps by reviewing the information in this chapter. If you get hurt, it will tell you what to do about it.

▶ **Chapter 4,** *Easy Exercises,* describes and illustrates 50 core fitness exercises. They are divided into three color-coded sections for easy reference: strength (blue), flexibility (green), and balance (orange). Each exercise comes with step-by-step instructions, and offers variations for beginners and older adults.

▶ **Chapter 5,** *The Workbook,* pulls everything together and outlines four weekly routines for you to follow for an all-around core fitness program. Are you also a golfer, runner, hiker, tennis player, bowler, swimmer, or work-in-the-yard exerciser? There is a core fitness program for you, too.

▶ **Appendix I:** *The Glossary* defines 44 fitness-related terms in easy-to-understand language.

▶ **Appendix II:** *Resources* is a list of 16 institutions and organizations where you can get more information.

Throughout this Special Report, look for sidebars titled *New Findings* and *Easy Tips*. They will inform you on the latest core fitness-related research and offer helpful suggestions to support your ongoing fitness.

1 THE CORE CONNECTION

Everything begins with the core. Whether you are sitting or standing as you read this report, you are using core muscles to maintain good posture. If you are slumping or slouching as you sit or stand, a weak or unbalanced core is probably the problem.

When you rise to a standing position, the core gets you started. When you stand, turn, bend, reach, twist, stoop, carry something, maintain your balance, walk, jog, swim, or participate in any physical activity, the action begins from the center of your body and moves out to your arms and legs (see Box 1-1, "Trunk muscle strength is associated with improved balance, daily functions, and prevention of falls"). Strength in the muscles of the arms and legs is necessary, but a strong core must support those muscles. When you decide to sit again, the core muscles help you land softly instead of flopping into a chair.

Weak or strong, core muscles affect almost everything you do during the day and a few movements you do at night—like turning over as you sleep or getting out of bed when you wake.

What is the core?

Exercise scientists have been inconsistent with their definitions of the core. Here are some examples:
▶ the underlying muscles of the torso
▶ every part of the body except the arms and legs
▶ the central link that connects your upper and lower body
▶ the muscles of the abdomen, lower back, and hips
▶ the pelvis, trunk, shoulders, and neck regions of the body

For the purposes of this report, we define the core as the muscles of the hips, pelvis, abdomen, and trunk. These core muscles have names that are scientific and not used in everyday conversations. Box 1-2, "The Abdominals," illustrates the location of four important core muscles, referred to as the "abs" (abdominals). When exercise instructions in Chapter 4 include the phrase "tighten your abs" or "tighten your stomach muscles," these are the ones to contract. All 10 core muscles are described in Box 1-3, "Core muscle name, location, and function."

These four abdominal muscles are used for protection, stability, bending, twisting, and posture:

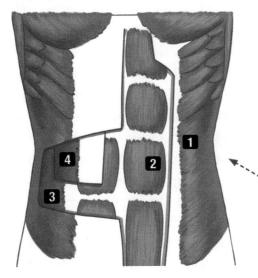

1 **External abdominal obliques:** Located on the side and front of the abdomen.

2 **Rectus abdominis:** Located along the front of the abdomen, this is the most well-known abdominal. Often referred to as the "six pack."

3 **Internal obliques:** Located under the external obliques, running in the opposite direction.

4 **Transverse abdominis:** Located under the obliques, it is the deepest of the abdominal muscles and wraps around your spine for protection and safety.

BOX 1-3

CORE MUSCLE NAME, LOCATION, AND FUNCTION

NAME	LOCATION	FUNCTION
Rectus abdominis	Abdomen	Flex/bend the trunk forward
Transverse abdominis	Abdomen	Support/stabilize the abdominal wall; posture
Internal obliques	Abdomen	Twist/rotate the trunk
External obliques	Sides	Twist/rotate the trunk
Multifidus	Back/spine	Extend/rotate/stabilize the spine
Spinal erectors	Back	Stand upright
Quadratus lumborum	Lower back	Flex the trunk to the sides; stabilize the pelvis
Gluteus maximus	Buttocks	Extend hips; rotate thighs; walk
Gluteus medius/ minimus	Buttocks	Rotate hips; stabilize pelvis; balance
Iliopsoas	Pelvis/hips	Rotate pelvis; bend at hips; stabilize the body while standing; balance

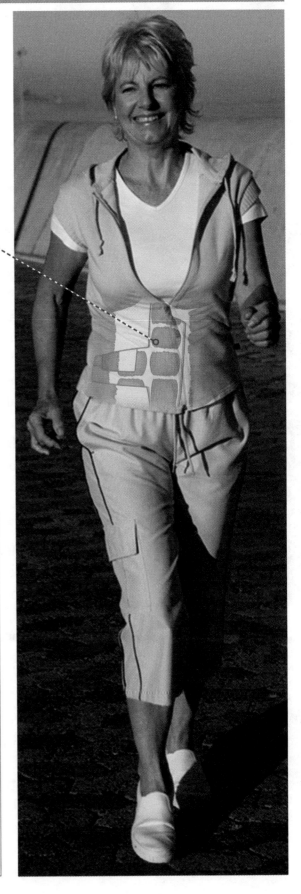

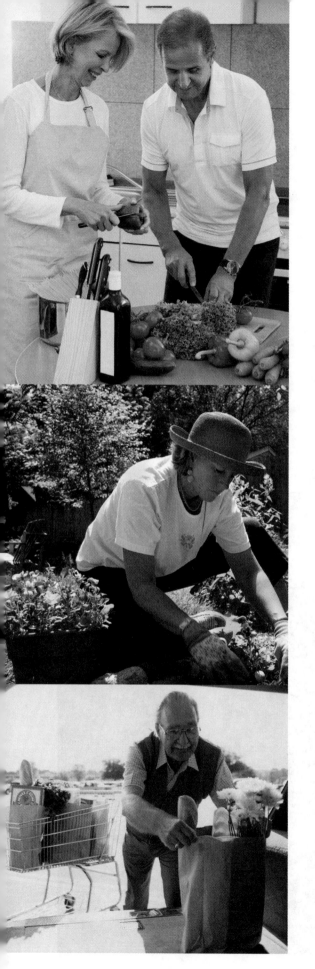

How the core affects daily activities

Core muscles stabilize segments of the body, act as a shock absorber for the whole body, maintain functional (working) posture, and allow for motions, such as flexion and rotation.

Each muscle and muscle group has a specific role to play in terms of daily activities.

Most of us don't think in terms of muscle names, their exact location, or their biomechanical functions, such as flexing, extending, rotating, or stabilizing. But when core muscles are weak, whether we notice it or not, they affect everyday acts. This includes activities like dressing, bathing, using a computer, sitting at a desk, carrying groceries, vacuuming, mopping, dusting, and participating in sports like golf, tennis, swimming, and biking.

Improving your core through regular resistance exercises can improve overall mobility. In fact, a study in the *Journal of the American Medical Association* showed that just moderate-intensity resistance exercise reduces disability and increases mobility among older adults (see Box 1-4, "Moderate-intensity exercise improves mobility").

As your mobility improves, and you can do more everyday chores, like housework and grocery shopping, you can reduce your risk of disability even further according to a Northwestern University study (see Box 1-5, "Light daily physical activity reduces disability").

Flexibility

Beyond simply allowing or supporting certain movements, the core is necessary for flexibility, strength, and injury prevention. Flexibility is the ability to move joints through a range of motion. Weak or tight muscles limit flexibility; strong muscles enhance it. Think of bending to pick up an object, stooping to do housework, dressing, or bathing.

In middle-aged and older adults, tight (less flexible) hamstrings and hip flexor muscles often affect muscles of the core, including those in the buttocks, pelvis, and lower back.

Strength

Strength is the ability to exert force against resistance. In a gym, that means lifting weights or pulling and pushing to move an object. At home, it's lifting a grandchild, carrying groceries, doing yard work, or in some cases, using your body weight as resistance—as in performing a modified push-up or getting through a day without being overly fatigued. Wherever it occurs, resistance training, often referred to as weight training, is the solution when lack of strength is the problem.

One of the strength-related obstacles older adults face is the loss of muscle mass. Sarcopenia—low muscle mass—affects as many as 50 percent of older adults, yet few people are familiar with the term. Decreased muscle strength and mass can lead to issues with mobility, frailty, osteoporosis, falls, pain, and fractures, as well as decreased activity, diabetes, and weight-gain. The accumulation of impairments can eventually result in the loss of physical function and independence. The risk of disability is up to 4.6 times higher in older persons with sarcopenia than in those with normal muscle tissue and strength.

One of the most basic interventions to offset the loss of muscle mass is resistance exercise designed to rebuild mass, strength, and performance (see Box 1-6, "Resistance training offsets the loss of muscle mass associated with aging," on the following page). The benefit of resistance training in this age group is effective only if it is combined with a nutrition program that includes adequate protein, fruits and vegetables, and vitamin D that lessens the impact of aging on muscle tissue (see "Muscle mass loss" on page 33).

Weakness in any part of the core may cause a person to overcompensate in other areas, which results in less efficient movement and an increased risk of pain or injury. The entire chain of movement can be disrupted if one link is weak or if a muscle or muscle group is overdeveloped. Overdevelopment can be associated with handedness—right-side muscles if the person is right-handed; left-side muscles if left-handed. It happens in others who may have strong abdominal muscles but weak muscles that support the lower back.

Flexibility and strength make participating in physical activities more enjoyable and safer. Both are helpful in skill sports, such as golf and tennis. They are equally important in activities as

NEW FINDING   BOX 1-4

Moderate-intensity exercise improves mobility

Participating in a daily moderate-intensity exercise program of aerobic, resistance, and flexibility activities is a feasible and effective intervention that reduces disability among older persons, according to researchers at the University of Florida and their colleagues across the country. More than 1,600 adults between the ages of 70 and 89 were randomly assigned to the exercise group or to a health education group, and their health was monitored for an average of 2.6 years. Those in the physical activity group were significantly more mobile at the end of the period than those in the health education only group, in spite of functional decline that occurs late in life.

Journal of the American Medical Association, May 2014

NEW FINDING   BOX 1-5

Light daily physical activity reduces disability

Performing light physical exercise, such as pushing a shopping cart or vacuuming, can help people avoid or delay disabilities associated with aging, according to researchers at Northwestern University. In what is believed to be the first study to show that exercise below the moderate and vigorous levels can help prevent disability, researchers monitored daily activities of 1,700 adults who wore accelerometers during waking hours for a week. Two years later, they completed surveys to determine the development of disabilities. As expected, those who participated in moderate and vigorous activities reported lower rates of disability. However, light intensity exercise was also related to fewer disabilities. The authors concluded that more time spent during the day simply moving may lower the risk of disability.

The BMJ, April 29, 2014

simple as walking or riding a bicycle (see Box 1-7, "Core strength improves spinal and functional mobility").

Injuries

Perhaps the most important practical application of core fitness is to guard against injuries. Low back pain, for example, affects as much as 80 percent of the population. Core muscles that support the spine may be the determining factor in whether you are included in that group. Chapter 3, "Preventing Injuries," contains detailed information about muscle strains, sprains, muscle imbalance, and cramps.

Falls/balance

Twenty percent of older adults have a problem with balance, and falls are a particular problem for people in that age group. The Centers for Disease Control and Prevention says that more than one-third of adults age 65 and older fall each year, and 20-30 percent of those suffer moderate to severe injuries. Strengthening core muscles is one way to guard against falls (see Box 1-8, "Exercise programs reduce the risk of falls and injuries caused by falls"). At least five of the 10 muscles listed in Box 1-3 on page 9 are directly related to balance, and the other five are indirectly related.

Signs that core muscles need work

The "abs" get most of the attention in advertisements for strength devices, and a big waist is something almost everyone tries to avoid. But the first sign of a weak core is poor posture—both standing and sitting. Other signs are back pain and muscle weakness.

Poor posture

The American Physical Therapy Association says that signs of poor posture include slouching, head thrusted or tilted forward, rounded shoulders, and excessive arching of the lower back (swayback). So, the body's natural curves are exaggerated. The opposite of poor posture is a position that minimizes strain on the joints and muscles.

The problem for most middle-aged and older adults is the difficulty in changing old posture habits. Knowing the checkpoints doesn't guarantee that a person can easily follow them. For that to happen, the core muscles have to be strengthened. Again, everything goes back to the core.

Lower back pain

A second indicator of a weak core is lower back pain. When unnecessary pressure is put on the vertebrae, discs, and facets that form the spinal column, back pain will let you know something is wrong with your posture. The appearance will be one of an excessive inward curvature of the lower spine and accompanying extension of the stomach/abdomen.

Weakness

The third weak-core warning signal is muscle weakness. You won't feel the weakness in your core, but rather in your arms and legs. A strong and stable core transfers strength that allows for rapid, strong, and efficient movement needed to lift, push, pull, throw, or stride.

What's next?

In Chapter 2, "Getting Ready," you'll learn the rules to follow for a safe core exercise program, become familiar with a few start-up terms (like *repetitions* and *sets*), get the information you need for warming up and cooling down, and most important, how to stick with a program once you've begun.

NEW FINDING   BOX 1-8

Exercise programs reduce the risk of falls and injuries caused by falls

Researchers in France reviewed 17 studies involving more than 4,000 subjects to determine if fall prevention exercise interventions are effective in preventing falls and fall-related injuries. They identified four categories of falls (all injurious falls, falls that resulted in medical care, severe injury falls, and falls that caused fractures) and found that exercise programs designed to prevent falls in older adults also prevented injuries caused by falls. In addition, the programs reduced the rate of falls that required medical care.

The BMJ, October 29, 2013

☑ EASY TIP

AVOID PROCRASTINATION
Plan for and schedule exercise. Don't wait until you have time or feel like it.

BOX 2-1

CHECKPOINTS FOR A NEUTRAL SPINE POSITION

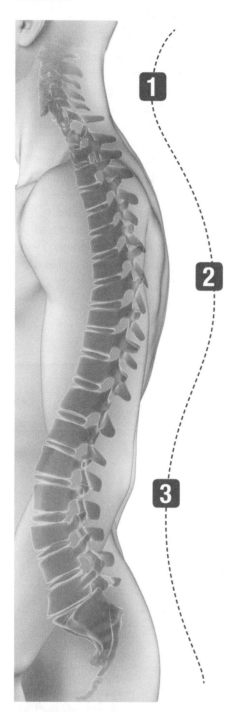

A neutral spine position has three natural curves:

1 **Cervical spine:** Neck, inward curve.

2 **Thoracic spine:** Middle of the back, outward curve.

3 **Lumbar spine:** Lower back, inward curve.

2 GETTING READY

Before you begin, you should be aware of guidelines that will make your workouts productive and safe. The suggestions that follow come from weight training experts, hospitals, universities, and organizations, including the American College of Sports Medicine.

1. Get the approval of your doctor before beginning an exercise program. Among the health issues that might restrict or prohibit a core fitness program are:
   - history of heart disease or respiratory conditions
   - current use of prescription medications
   - surgery or bone/muscle/tendon/ligament problems that might be aggravated by exercise
   - any other related health or physical issue
   - a previously sedentary lifestyle among females age 50 and older and males age 40 and older

2. Wear comfortable, loose-fitting nylon clothing that wicks moisture (perspiration) away from your body.

3. Wear properly fitted athletic shoes that provide traction and lateral support. Also wear dry-fit socks to avoid blisters and chafing.

4. Use proper technique. If you are not sure how to perform an exercise, get a physical therapist or athletic trainer to teach you.

5. Maintain good posture by keeping a neutral spine position. A natural-curve, neutral spine position is described and illustrated in Box 2-1, "Checkpoints for a neutral spine position."

6. Vary your exercise routine and seek a balance between muscle groups—left side/right side or front/back.

7. Don't hold your breath. Breathe out as you lift; breathe in as you lower a weight.

8. Develop a workout tempo. Don't jerk or move quickly. Stay in control.

9. Listen to your body. If something hurts, stop, and try it again a few days later.

10. Stay hydrated by drinking plenty of water before, during, and after exercise.

11. Give your body time to recover after vigorous exercise—48 hours between core fitness workouts that involve the same muscle group.

What is a repetition (rep)?

A repetition, or rep—the number of times you perform an exercise.

What is a set?

A set is a group or series of the same kind of exercise. For example, one set of five modified push-up includes doing five pushups before stopping.

How much is enough?

Use a weight or other type of resistance you can lift, push, pull, or move 8-12 times while using good form. Complete one set of 8-12 repetitions before resting when you are beginning a program, then add 2-3 sets as you get stronger and more accustomed to the workout. Gradually, add resistance (2-3 pounds) when you can perform 12 reps in two consecutive sets with good form.

How often?

Perform core resistance-training exercises 3-4 non-consecutive days per week.

Good exercise technique includes using the right amount of weight and resting between sets.

Technique matters

The illustrations in Chapter 4 show the correct form for 50 core exercises. But technique involves more than correct form. Consider the speed of movement it takes to perform an exercise, the range of motion through which your muscles and joints should move, and how you should breathe while doing the activity. Box 2-2, "Core exercise technique tips," is a quick-reference guide.

BOX 2-2

Core exercise technique tips

☑ **Speed of movement:** Approximately 6 seconds per repetition.

☑ **Range of motion:** Full range, from full stretch to complete contraction.

☑ **Breathing:** Exhale when lifting a weight. Inhale when lowering a weight.

☑ **Rest between sets:** 30-90 seconds, depending on intensity of the lift.

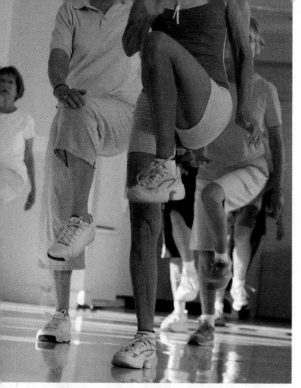

It's important to warm up before exercise by gradually elevating your heart rate and raising your body's temperature.

NEW FINDING   BOX 2-3

Foam rollers ease muscle fatigue and soreness

Foam rollers, once considered an exercise gimmick, are now a standard piece of equipment used during exercise warm ups. Twenty-six men and women were tested to measure the effects of using foam rollers and a planking exercise during a warm up before a series of athletic performances (jumping, isometric force, and agility). There were no significant differences between foam roller use and planking on the athletic tests, but there was significantly less fatigue and soreness from pre- to post-exercise for both kinds of exercise. Post-exercise fatigue after foam rolling was significantly less than after the subjects performed planking exercises. The study strengthens the case for using foam rollers as part of a warm up routine.

Journal of Strength and Conditioning Research, January 2014

Warm up

Rule number one: Don't stretch first. Warm up to loosen up. The quickest way to strain a cold muscle or muscle group is to stretch it as far as you can before doing any physical activity. Save "static" stretches for your "cool down" after your exercise session.

Instead, do something to gradually elevate your heart rate, increase blood circulation, raise your body's temperature, and perhaps even break a sweat.

Get a head start on warming up by taking a sauna, a warm shower, or use warm, moist wraps or towels, or a heating pad to ease joint stiffness and raise body temperature. A light jog, walk, or gentle calisthenics can achieve the same effect.

Foam rollers have also been shown to loosen and warm up muscle tissue and "work the knots out" (see Box 2-3, "Foam rollers ease muscle fatigue and soreness"). They are inexpensive and work as a self-massage. The medical term for this task is myofascial release.

Another way to warm up is the least technical and most practical. It is called ballistic stretching, but it means using the motions you will employ during an exercise or activity, but at a slower, easier pace. For example, if you are going to perform "wall push-ups" as part of your core exercise routine, go through the wall push-up motion standing closer to the wall, moving slower, and doing fewer repetitions than you will eventually do during the session.

You also can use this type of warm up when you get ready for a sport or for aerobic exercise. Warm up for tennis by hitting easy groundstrokes from a position in the middle of the court. Get ready for a round of golf by taking easy swings on the driving range. Warm up for a walk by walking slowly at first, then gradually increase the pace.

Cool down

After an exercise session, don't just walk away. Take a few minutes to cool down. It will reduce the risk of blood pooling in your legs, avoid the risk of a sudden drop in blood pressure, and allow your pulse to return to normal in a controlled manner. Some exercise physiologists say to cool down until your pulse rate drops below 100 beat per minute. The better your physical condition, the sooner your pulse will return to its normal rate.

Now is when you can stretch. There is evidence that static stretching at the end of exercise increases range of motion in subsequent sessions. Stretch the same muscles used during your exercise program. The rules for static stretching:

- Begin slowly
- Hold the stretch for about 30 seconds
- Don't bounce
- Perform six to eight stretches per session
- Perform two to three repetitions per stretch
- Don't forget to breathe

Sticking with the program

The hardest part of increasing and maintaining core fitness will be making it a permanent part of your daily or weekly routine. According to a recent study, about one-half of older adults who get into an exercise group drop out before it has been completed (see Box 2-4, "Half of exercise program participants drop out"). Another study found that factors, such as goal setting, exercise adherence contracts, instructor feedback, and self-monitoring, may be beneficial in encouraging adults to stay with a program (see Box 2-5, "Goal setting and instructor feedback help participants adhere to an exercise program").

You are less likely to be a dropout if your exercise program is:

- **Scheduled:** instead of exercising when you have time
- **Enjoyable:** something you look forward to doing
- **Convenient:** conducted at a location near your home
- **Conducted with others:** instead of exercising alone
- **Challenging:** works all of the major core muscles
- **Measurable:** in terms of compliance or gains in strength, flexibility, and balance

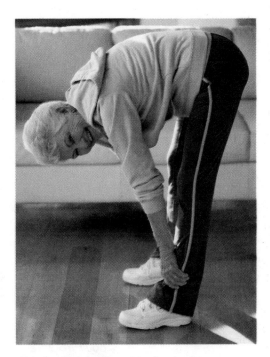

Always stretch after exercise and never before. Evidence suggests that stretching at the end of a session increases range of motion in future workouts.

NEW FINDING   BOX 2-4

Half of exercise program participants drop out

Only one-half of older women adhere to programs of aerobic and resistance training exercise programs, according to a recent study. More than 200 women with an average age of 70 enrolled in a program of regular exercise designed to minimize the physical decline associated with aging. Of those in the aerobic exercise group, 49.7 percent completed the program. Fifty-six percent completed the strength training program. Multiple factors, including motivation, were associated with adherence to both programs.

Clinical Interventions in Aging, February 14, 2014

NEW FINDING   BOX 2-5

Goal setting and instructor feedback help participants adhere to an exercise program

Sixty-three adults with an average age 63.8 were assigned to either 1) a six-week exercise group followed by a five-week program in which motivational strategies were added; 2) an exercise-only program; or 3) a control group. The motivational components for the experimental group were instituted at various stages of the program. The research team found that interventions, such as goal setting, exercise contracts, instructor feedback, self-monitoring, and exercise, may be beneficial in motivating older adults to adhere to an exercise program.

Current Gerontology and *Geriatrics Research,* December 2013

Equipment options

Some people are reluctant to begin an exercise because they think sophisticated machines or expensive gym equipment are needed. Not so with core fitness. The core can be strengthened using body-weight exercises—using your own body as resistance—or easy-to-use items like stability balls, free weights, medicine balls, resistance bands, and even chairs.

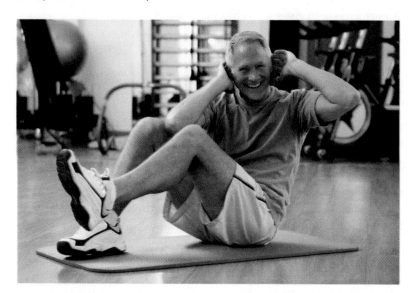

Modified sit-ups are an example of using your body weight to strengthen your core muscles.

Body weight

The classic examples of body weight exercises are pull-ups, standard sit-ups and push-ups, although those three exercises are not necessarily recommended options for core strengthening. Better examples of exercises for using body weight for core strengthening are modified sit-ups, wall push-ups, and semi-sits (see workbook section, beginning on page 38).

Stability balls

Stability balls, also referred to as physioballs and gymnastic balls, have become a mainstream piece of equipment for stretching and strengthening core-related muscles. They can be used instead of a bench for traditional strength exercises. Sitting on a stability ball and gently bouncing engages muscles of the legs, abdomen, and back. The instability of the ball forces a person to use his or her core muscles to keep the body level.

Stability balls come in different sizes. When sitting on the ball, your thighs should be parallel to the floor. Box 2-6, "Choosing the right size stability ball," gives general guidelines for the appropriate size of the ball according to an individual's height.

A highly inflated ball makes it unstable and thus requires more

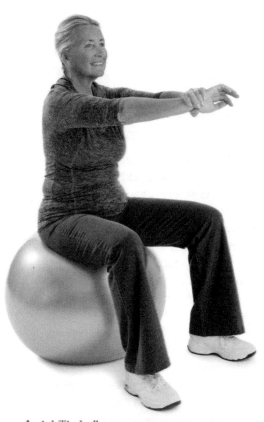

A stability ball can engage many core muscles as well as the legs and back.

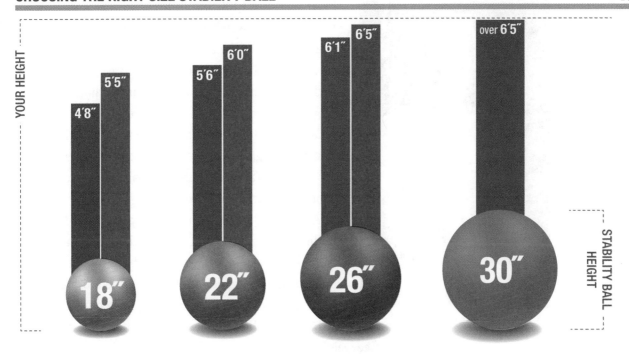

effort; less air is better and safer for beginners and intermediates. Maintain a wide leg spread when doing stability ball exercises and always have a spotter to help prevent loss of balance and falls.

Stability balls also can be used along with other equipment to enhance the exercise. For instance, sitting on a stability ball while using a free weight is an example of combining one type of exercise (free weights) with another (stability ball). Together, they engage core muscles to a higher degree than doing the same exercise on a stable surface.

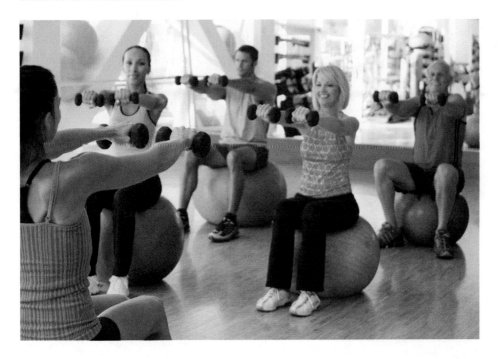

☑ **EASY TIP**

DON'T DO TOO MUCH TOO SOON
Gradually increase the number of repetitions, sets, and intensity (never more than 10 percent of the previous week's workout).

Combining two types of exercise equipment, like performing free weights on a stability ball, engages multiple core muscles in a single movement.

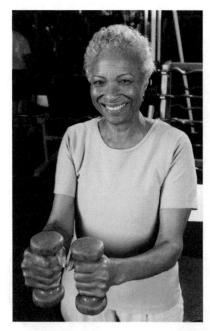

Hand-held free weights are a staple exercise equipment.

Free weights (dumbbells)

Hand-held free weights, or dumbbells, are thought of as weights for the arms or legs. For beginning exercisers and older adults, two-to-three pounds in each hand is enough to lift, but many seniors quickly move up to those that weigh between five and eight pounds. Very light weights require more repetitions to gain strength. Heavier dumbbells require fewer repetitions to achieve the same goals, but be careful about too much weight too soon.

A free weight doesn't have to be a purchased either. A filled, plastic water bottle weighs between one and two pounds, can be held easily, and can substitute for a dumbbell. A one-gallon milk carton filled (or partially filled) that has a handle serves the same purpose, and you may have other household objects that can substitute for free weights.

See page 43 for exercises using free weights.

Chair-based exercises

Chair-based exercises can be just the right choice for those who need extra support because of lack of strength or mobility. A secure comfortable chair can be used as a substitute for almost any exercise that requires standing or sitting on a stability ball, and can help you safely and effectively perform many core-building movements until your strength and endurance improves. This concept was recently confirmed by researchers in the United Kingdom and published in *BMC Geriatrics* (see Box 2-7, "Chair-based exercise develops core strength").

Resistance bands are a low-cost fitness tool that can be used for a variety of core exercises.

Resistance bands

Resistance bands and tubes offer a versatile, inexpensive, and space-saving option. They provide an appealing convenience factor. A wide range of movements can be performed at home, at work, or in a hotel room. Exercises include curls, shrugs, partial squats, and leg swings.

Pharmacies and medical supply stores

sell resistance bands in rolls that can be cut to desired lengths, as well as in pre-determined lengths. Some have handle attachments; with others you can simply wrap the ends around your hands. The bands are also color-coded to correspond with light, medium, and heavy resistance. Prices range from $7 to $25.

However, resistance bands have their limitations. They wear out with age and use. The amount of resistance is hard to measure, there is a lack of uniform resistance throughout the range of movement, and the color codes differ from company to company. Check them often for nicks and tears, and avoid storing them in extremely hot or cold temperatures. Remove your rings before an exercise session and avoid objects or surfaces that could cause a tear. Depending on use, resistance bands should be replaced every three to four months.

See pages 41-42 and 46 for exercises using resistance bands.

Medicine balls

Medicine balls (med-balls) are versatile workout equipment that can be incorporated into other many forms of training. They can help develop speed, power, and balance. Traditional med-ball workouts consisted primarily of abdominal exercises, but now they include exercises for the arms, shoulders, back, chest, and legs.

Medicine balls are available in weights that range from two to 30 pounds. The goal is to use a weight that is challenging for the number of repetitions a person attempts to complete. Having several balls of varying weights allows for a variety of exercises and differences in exercise intensity.

Medicine balls are not designed to focus on developing strength. Instead, they are used to convert strength into dynamic movement. They might be helpful in increasing power for hitting a golf ball or swinging a tennis racket, but not so much for increasing muscle size or strength.

See pages 45, 48-49, 53 for exercises using medicine balls.

Chair-based exercise develops core strength

A group of physicians and exercise scientists in the United Kingdom conducted a review of literature and confirmed that chair-based exercises (CBE) are an appropriate form of resistance and flexibility training for older or frail adults. Among the findings:

1. The purpose of using a chair is to promote stability in both sitting and standing;

2. CBE should be considered as part of a continuum of exercise in which progression is encouraged; and

3. CBE should be used as a starting point to progress to standing programs.

BMC Geriatrics, May 19, 2014

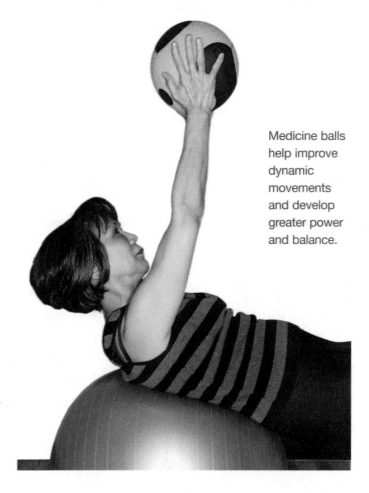

Medicine balls help improve dynamic movements and develop greater power and balance.

Yoga, tai chi, and Pilates

These three mind-body modalities help improve balance and coordination. You may be familiar with one or even all three, as they are offered at most fitness clubs and recreational centers. They each offer different levels of intensity and modifications so you can adjust to meet your fitness level and physical limitations. All three are ideal programs to supplement the basic core fitness programs presented in this report. Here is a more detailed look at each one and what they can offer:

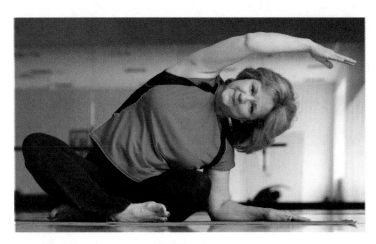

Yoga is offered in many styles and can complement other exercise routines.

Yoga

Yoga uses movement, meditation, relaxation, and gentle breathing, all of which contribute to a sense of self-awareness. For some people, yoga is a spiritual experience; for others it is an alternative exercise that promotes flexibility, strength, and endurance.

According to a National Health Interview Survey, more than 13 million adults in the U.S. practiced yoga during the previous year. The Mayo Clinic says that practicing yoga can lead to improved balance, flexibility, range of motion, and strength, and that most people can benefit from a variety of yoga styles.

The National Center for Complementary and Alternative Medicine (NCCAM) says yoga may help reduce pain and improve function. It is usually low-impact and safe for healthy people when practiced appropriately under the guidance of a well-trained instructor. One NCCAM-funded study of people with chronic low-back pain found that yoga resulted in significantly less disability, pain, and depression after six months. Conclusions from another study of adults with chronic or recurring low-back pain suggested that 12 weekly yoga classes resulted in better function than usual medical care.

The NCCAM provides these guidelines for considering yoga as a form of exercise or therapy:

- Do not use yoga to replace conventional medical care.
- If you have a medical condition, talk with your doctor before joining a yoga class.
- Ask one of your health care providers to recommend a yoga instructor.
- Carefully consider the type of yoga you choose to practice.
- Tell your health care providers about yoga or any other health practices you use.

Tai chi

More than two million Americans participate in individual or group tai chi sessions each year, according to the National Health Interview Survey. Studies have confirmed that tai chi can improve balance, overcome a fear of falling, lower the risk of falls, reduce blood pressure, and provide a general sense of well-being. It is especially effective in older adults because it can be practiced at different intensity levels.

Tai chi is a combination of relaxation, meditation, deep breathing, and slow, gentle, continuous, and structured exercises called forms. It is said to achieve harmony between body and mind. The number of movements range from 18 to more than 100. Newcomers begin with as little as one, five-minute session per week and gradually increase to a higher target goal. Finding a qualified instructor can be a challenge because certification has not been standardized.

Tai chi appears to be safe and effective, but people with the following conditions should get the advice of a physician before beginning a program:

- osteoporosis
- chest pain with minimal exertion
- severe shortness of breath
- dizziness or fainting spells
- uncontrolled blood pressure
- gait and balance disorders

The slow, gentle movements of tai chi help improve balance and coordination.

Pilates

Pilates is generally recognized as a method of building strength in core muscles for better posture, balance, and flexibility. It has also been used as a way to treat and prevent back pain. The NCCAM describes it as movement therapy that uses a method of physical

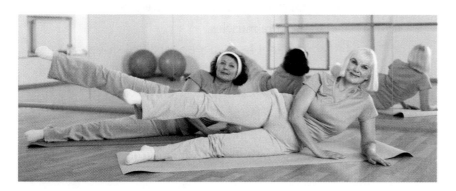

Pilates is a floor-based exercise that emphasizes core muscles.

BOX 2-8

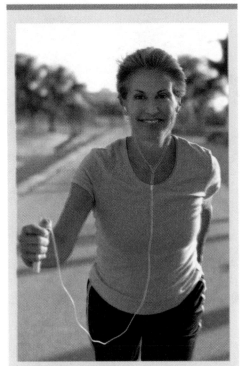

Proper walking techniques

- Head up, eyes forward, chin parallel to the ground.
- Shoulders relaxed and down, but not hunched.
- Back neither arched nor slumped.
- Elbows slightly bent, arms swinging front to back, not side to side.

☑ **EASY TIP**

ALWAYS START BY WARMING UP
Take 5-10 minutes to loosen muscle tissue, increase circulation, and break a light sweat.

exercise to strengthen and build control of muscles, especially those used for posture.

Pilates consists of 25 to 50 low-impact strength and endurance movements. Many of the exercises can be performed on a floor or mat. As with other exercise programs, talk with your doctor before beginning a Pilates program. It is not recommended or should be modified for people who have unstable blood pressure, a risk of blood clots, severe osteoporosis, or a herniated disc.

Walking

Walking is one of the easiest exercises available. All you need is a pair of fitted comfortable shoes and a safe terrain on which to walk. You can do it almost anywhere—from around your neighborhood to a gym treadmill. Walking is an ideal workout for people who are beginning a fitness program, returning to exercise after a long layoff, or recovering from an injury. In terms of core fitness, walking is a great means to warm up and cool down the body for each designed workout program. Always make sure to follow healthy walking posture (see Box 2-8, "Proper walking techniques").

Testing for core fitness

As mentioned throughout this report, you should not engage in any new or demanding physical activity, exercise, or test without getting the approval of your doctor. Signs of core weakness, such as poor posture, muscle weakness, and low back pain are easy for most people to assess without a professional. But a physician, physical therapist, exercise physiologist, strength coach, or athletic trainer is needed to provide a more scientific evaluation.

Among the tests used specifically for older adults are the Senior Fitness Test, the AAHPERD Functional Fitness Test, and the Groningen Fitness Test. Each one tests core strength, flexibility, balance, and mobility, all of which are directly or indirectly related to the core muscles.

Three tests that might be used are a modified sit-up, a "functional reach" assessment, and an "excursion balance" test. In one study, each of those tests was used to evaluate core strength and its effect on balance in a group of subjects between the ages of 65 and 85 (see Box 2-9, "Core muscle strength improves balance"). Improvements in core muscle endurance were associated with significant improvements in balance.

Self-test

The 30-second sit-to-stand chair test, starting from a seated position, is an indirect test of core strength, a direct test of leg strength and endurance, and a predictor of risk for falls, according to Centers for Disease Control and Prevention. It is also an exercise you can do at home (assuming you have your doctor's permission) to improve lower body and core strength.

The exercise requires a sturdy chair that has a straight back and no arms, a stopwatch, and someone to act as a spotter and timer. With arms folded across your chest, complete as many sit-to-stand repetitions as you can in 30 seconds (see Box 2-10, "30-second sit-to-stand chair test," on the following page). A below average score indicates a high risk for falls.

Good posture

Maintaining good posture when you stand and sit is also necessary to ensure your can safely practice some of the core muscle movements in the exercise programs. A change in posture is as much mental as it is physical. It's one thing to sit up straight or stand tall for the moment, but quite another to strengthen and train your muscles to support good posture on a long-term basis.

Try two mental exercises to increase posture awareness whether standing, walking, or sitting. The first is "rising like a balloon"— thinking about good posture in vertical terms, energy that flows upward, and becomes lighter. The second is aligning your head over your shoulders as though a string is pulling on it from above. When the head is up, the body finds the most efficient way to support it, and the result is good, comfortable posture.

Box 2-11, "Standing and sitting posture checklist," is a point-by-point checklist for standing and sitting postures. It's best to have someone else observe your posture and compare it to the checklist.

Core muscle strength improves balance

At the University of Toledo, researchers enlisted a group of 24 men and women between the ages of 65 and 85 to determine the effect of core muscle strengthening on balance. The participants were assigned to an experimental exercise group or a control group. The exercise group performed a core-strengthening home program three times a week for six weeks that consisted of a modified sit-up, a functional reaching exercise, and a balance activity. The experimental group showed significant improvements in all three tests compared with those in the control group. The results suggested core strengthening should be a part of a comprehensive balance training program for older adults.

Journal of Aging & Physical Activity, January, 2014

BOX 2-11

Standing and sitting posture checklist

CORRECT STANDING POSTURE		CORRECT SITTING POSTURE	
☑ **Head:** Up, not forward, backward, or sideways	☑ **Abdomen:** In	☑ **Back:** Straight	☑ **Knees:** Bent at a right angle
	☑ **Lower back:** Normal curve	☑ **Shoulders:** Back and relaxed	☑ **Feet:** Flat on the floor
☑ **Shoulders:** Relaxed and back, but not too far back	☑ **Knees:** Relaxed, not locked	☑ **Buttocks:** Touching the back of the chair	
☑ **Chest:** Held high	☑ **Feet:** Parallel, weight balanced evenly	☑ **Weight:** Evenly distributed on both hips	

30-SECOND SIT-TO-STAND CHAIR TEST

BOX 2-10

▶ Sit in the middle of a sturdy chair, feet flat on the floor.

▶ Cross your arms. Keep your back straight, arms against your chest.

▶ Rise to a full standing position and then sit back down again.

▶ Repeat as many times as you can in 30 seconds.

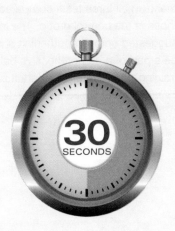

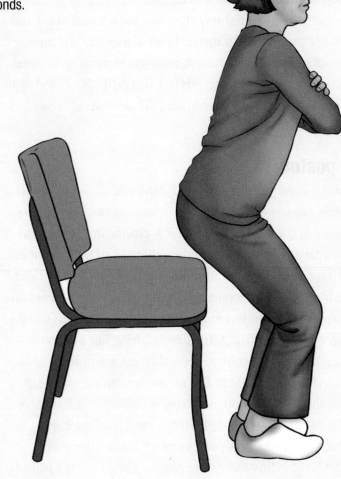

Record your score in the box, below.

Compare your score to the scores on right.

30-second chair stand test: Below average scores*

AGE	60-64	65-69	70-74	75-79	80-84	85-89	90-94
MEN	< 14	< 12	< 12	< 11	< 10	< 8	< 7
WOMEN	< 12	< 11	< 10	< 10	< 9	< 8	< 4

*Below average score indicates high risk for falls.

It's never too late

The benefits of exercise go far beyond good posture, getting through daily activities without being worn out, avoiding low back pain, and preventing falls. The average person loses between five and seven pounds of muscle tissue during every decade of adult life. The result is a cycle of reduced function, less physical activity, and further muscle loss.

Exercising the core and other muscle groups can stop and even reverse that cycle and lead to better function, more physical activity, and increased muscle tissue.

And it's never too late to start. One study showed that two months of strength training produced 3.7 additional pounds of muscle tissue in older, sedentary men; 1.7 pounds more muscle in women. Both groups achieved their results through 30-minute training sessions two-three days a week.

There are other benefits too, including:

- better weight control
- increased bone mineral density
- lower risk of some cancers
- improved blood lipid levels
- decreased low back pain
- better balance
- reduced body fat
- lower blood pressure
- lower risk of type 2 diabetes
- less pain from arthritis
- improved mood and mental health
- reduced risk of falling

Improving core fitness could be the start of something big. When core muscles get stronger, better flexibility and balance are sure to follow. Core fitness plus a sensible program of aerobic exercise and nutrition will improve the quality of your life and may even help you live longer.

What's next?

Before you being a regular exercise program to build and maintain core fitness, you need to ensure you can properly take care of your body. This includes how to prevent and treat common injuries and practice good nutrition.

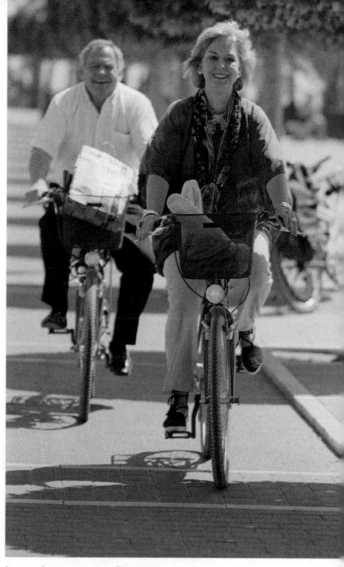

Improving your core fitness can make many everyday activities more enjoyable.

☑ **EASY TIP**

STRETCH AFTER, NOT BEFORE, EXERCISING

Warm up, go through the motions of the exercise to be performed, but at a slower, easier pace, and stretch after the workout.

☑ **EASY TIP**

DON'T SKIP COOLING DOWN

Take a few minutes after a workout to get your pulse and body temperature back to normal by walking, stretching, or slowing down in some other way.

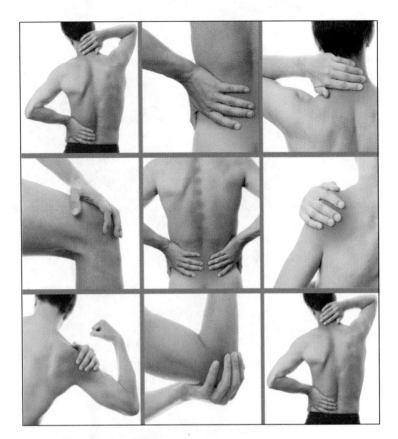

Muscle strain, sprains, and cramps can be common ailments when exercising and affect the major joints and muscle areas.

3 PREVENTING INJURIES

A risk-reward factor exists between exercise and injuries, but the rewards are far greater than the risks. They range from short-term benefits like feeling better immediately after an exercise session and helping in weight control to long-term gains, such as improved quality of life and longer life expectancy. The risk is mostly short-term—sustaining a musculoskeletal injury that, while painful or inconvenient, is treatable and not life changing. Three of the most common are strains, sprains, and cramps.

Strains

Most people use the term "pulled muscle" instead of "muscle strain" when they have stretched or torn a muscle or tendon. Tendons connect muscles to bones. Strains can occur anywhere a muscle-tendon unit is housed, including the shoulders, neck, abdominal area, back, hip, and upper legs (quadriceps and hamstrings)—all directly or indirectly connected to the body's core. People who have an increased risk of pulled muscles are those who have a history of strains, those who are overweight, and those in poor physical condition.

See Box 3-1, "Muscle strains: Causes, treatment, and prevention," for an overview.

Below are the five most common immediate causes of strains:

1. **Overexertion/Overuse:** too many repetitions of a physical activity
2. **Not warming up properly:** exercising vigorously before increasing body temperature and circulation
3. **Sudden or unusual movements:** jerking a weight or moving quickly during an activity, slipping, lifting a heavy weight, or lifting in an awkward position

4. **Fatigue:** exercising for long periods or not allowing for proper recovery time between exercise sessions

5. **Nutritional deficiencies:** cramps, for example

Symptoms

Symptoms include sudden pain, soreness, limited range of movement, bruising or discoloration, swelling, muscle spasms, stiffness, or weakness. Strains are classified according to the amount of damage sustained. Grade 1 strains involve a stretched muscle-tendon unit. Grade 2 strains mean a partial tear in muscle tissue has occurred. In Grade 3, the unit is completely torn.

Treatment

If you sustain a muscle strain, the initial home treatment is

1. Rest (24-48 hours)
2. Cold/ice pack applications (15-20 minutes, three or four times a day, two hours between cold packs)
3. Compression with an elastic bandage (but not too tight) when practical
4. Elevation (which may be impractical because of the location of some core muscles)

Over-the-counter medications (aspirin, ibuprofen, naproxen) can ease the discomfort and initial swelling. If there is significant swelling, pain, fever, bleeding, or inability to walk or move, seek immediate medical attention.

Once you resume physical activity following a strain, take it easy. Gradually work up to the exercise frequency, intensity, and duration you were able to do before the injury. Applying heat before exercise (a warm shower or warm, moist compresses) increases circulation and loosen muscle tissue. Ice applications after exercise help control swelling and reduce the pain.

Prevention: 10 tips

Here are 10 tips to reduce the risk of muscle strains:

1. Participate in a conditioning program to build muscle strength.
2. Perform stretching exercises daily (after warming up).
3. Wear shoes that fit and provide support (as opposed to simply feeling comfortable; get professionally fitted at a specialized running store).

BOX 3-1

Muscle strains: Causes, treatment, and prevention

☑ **Causes**
- Overexertion
- Overuse
- Not warming up
- Sudden movement
- Fatigue
- Not cooling down

☑ **Treatment**
- Protection
- Rest
- Ice first; heat later
- Compression
- Elevation
- Pain medications

☑ **Prevention**
- Strength training
- Stretching after warm ups
- Shoes that support movement
- Nutrition that supports exercise
- Avoid sitting in one position
- Use chair that supports lower back
- Know your limits

☑ **EASY TIP**

CHANGE YOUR EXERCISE ROUTINE
Vary your program to engage other muscles and muscle groups, and to prevent getting bored.

BOX 3-2

Sprains: Causes, treatments, and prevention

☑ **Causes**

- Forcing a joint beyond normal range of motion

☑ **Treatment**

- Protection
- Rest
- Ice first, heat later

☑ **Prevention**

- Strength training
- Flexibility training
- Shoes that provide lateral support

☑ **EASY TIP**

SET REALISTIC GOALS

Don't expect instant results! Set exercise goals that are a slight challenge, yet reachable. Once reached, set new goals. Incorporating exercise is a lifestyle change.

4. Nourish muscles by eating a well-balanced diet and drinking plenty of water.
5. Warm up before any physical activity, including resistance, aerobic, and flexibility training, as well as sports.
6. Stretch after exercise to prevent stiffness.
7. Use or wear protective equipment for each activity, when necessary.
8. Avoid sitting in one position for long periods of time.
9. Use a chair that provides good support for the lower back.
10. Know your limits. Build strength and flexibility gradually, and don't overdo it.

Sprains

Sprains are less likely to happen during core exercises than muscles strains, but they remain one of the most common types of injuries. A sprain occurs when a joint is forced beyond its normal range of motion. For instance, one or more of the ligaments that hold the bones of that joint together have been over-stretched, partially torn, or ruptured. It could happen to any joint, but ankles and knees are the most common sites. The ligaments most likely to be sprained run along the outside of the ankle. Up to 80 percent of all ankle sprains happen when the foot rolls toward the outside of the ankle. An awkward step or bad landing is all it takes.

Symptoms

As with strains, sprains are classified according to the amount of damage. Grade 1 sprains cause mild pain, localized swelling, and tenderness, but the ankle or knee remains stable and is not bruised. The ligaments are stretched but not torn.

With Grade 2 sprains, you may hear a popping or tearing sound when the ankle rolls to the side or the knee moves awkwardly. There is noticeable bruising, and internal bleeding will occur, which might not be observed for three or four days. Tenderness, swelling, limited range of motion, and difficulty walking are common. The ligament has been torn, but the ankle or knee could show signs of instability.

In Grade 3 sprains, the pain is severe, the swelling and tenderness are obvious, and the ankle or knee is unstable. Walking is difficult, if not impossible, and the person might feel that the ankle or knee will give way, and with good reason: the ligament has been significantly or completely torn.

See Box 3-2, "Sprains: Causes, treatment, and prevention," for an overview.

Treatment

Depending on the severity, follow the same protocol as with sprains. Stay off the ankle (or other joint) for 24-48 hours; apply an ice bag for 15 minutes, four times a day with a couple of hours between applications; compress the joint with an elastic wrap; protect it with an air brace or similar support; and elevate it at least two or three hours a day. Over-the-counter pain medications reduce pain, and aspirin and ibuprofen minimize pain and inflammation. It is important not to immobilize a joint that has been sprained for a long time. The longer it is immobilized, the weaker the muscles supporting the joint become and the longer it will take to return to normal.

Prevention

Some sprains are inevitable, but others might be prevented through a strength and flexibility exercise routine. Flexibility of the Achilles tendon is especially important to withstand the forces placed on it by strenuous activity. Shoes that provide lateral support also may help. Remember that a past sprain is the most common predictor of a future sprain, so building strength and increasing flexibility is even more important once you have been injured.

Cramps

Muscle cramps are sudden, involuntary, and painful muscle contractions. The lower leg is often affected. The exact cause is not known and the reasons appear to vary from person to person. Contributing factors are hot and humid weather, vigorous exercise, sweating, fatigue, dehydration, and possible deficiencies in minerals, such as calcium, sodium, and magnesium (also referred to as electrolytes). When these minerals are depleted, muscles may not contract properly. The regular use of diuretics can interfere with the body's mineral balance and contribute to cramping.

See Box 3-3, "Cramps: Causes, treatment, and prevention," for an overview.

BOX 3-3

Cramps: Causes, treatment, and prevention

☑ **Causes**
- Fatigue
- Prolonged exertion
- Electrolyte depletion
- Dehydration

☑ **Treatment**
- Stretching
- Ice applications
- Pressure
- Massage
- Fluids

☑ **Prevention**
- Improved fitness
- Stretching
- Warm up, cool down
- Hydration
- Eat more fruits, vegetables
- Massage
- No high heels
- Shoes that support exercise

More muscle mass in older adults reduces the risk of dying prematurely

Research at the David Geffen School of Medicine at UCLA suggests that increased muscle mass is associated with less likelihood of dying prematurely. Data from more than 3,600 men and women, ages 55 and older and 65 and older, respectively, at the time of the original survey, was used to determine how many individuals had died from natural causes during a follow-up time period ranging from 10 to 16 years. Body composition and body mass index (BMI) was measured periodically during the time period using bioelectrical impedance. All-cause mortality was significantly lower in the fourth quartile of muscle mass index (the highest category) when compared with those in the first quartile (lowest category). The study adds to a growing body of evidence that body composition is a better predictor of mortality than BMI and suggests clinicians should focus on ways to improve body composition rather than body mass index alone.

American Journal of Medicine, online March 13, 2014

☑ **EASY TIP**

DON'T NEGLECT BALANCE EXERCISES

Complete exercise programs involve resistance training, aerobic exercise, flexibility, and balance training, especially for older adults.

Treatment

Stretching, massage, and ice applications are three of the most common treatment strategies for cramps. If cramps are an ongoing problem or if they last longer than a few minutes, see your doctor.

Prevention

▶ Increase your level of fitness

▶ Include stretching in your core fitness routine

▶ Warm up before and cool down after exercise

▶ Drink water before, during, and after exercise, and stay hydrated even on days you do not exercise

▶ Include plenty of fruits and vegetables in your diet

▶ Consider massage as a method to reduce muscle tension

▶ Avoid high heels and wear shoes that provide comfort and support

Muscle imbalance

Muscle imbalance is as complex as it is common. Muscles and muscle groups are supposed to work together for strength, flexibility, balance, posture, and movement. Biceps and triceps alternately contract to allow the elbows to bend. Deltoids and lattisimus dorsi raise and lower the arms. Abdominal muscles and back muscles that support the spine allow us to bend forward and backward. Hip abductors and adductors move the legs closer together or farther apart. And the quadriceps on the front of the upper legs depend on the hamstrings (on the back sides of the upper leg) to help us bend and straighten our knees.

For a variety of reasons, imbalances exist and the result is inefficient movement, poor posture, and susceptibility to injuries and muscular conditions. Knee pain, low back pain, and Achilles tendinitis are three of many examples. The simplest way to improve muscle imbalance is to choose exercises that strengthen opposing muscle groups.

How do you know?

Muscle imbalance is often easy to recognize. Repeated injuries that involve the same muscle groups or same side of the body are one way. Poor standing, walking, or sitting posture are others. But you may need professional help to identify and resolve a muscle imbalance problem. A licensed physical or occupational therapist (PT or OT), an athletic trainer (AT or ATC), or a certified strength and conditioning specialist (CSCS) can give you an accurate assessment, as well as recommend exercises to address the problem.

Longevity

The greatest long-term benefit of exercise appears to be longevity. Recent research at UCLA suggests that increased muscle mass is associated with less likelihood of dying prematurely and that body composition is a better indicator of mortality than standard measurements like body mass index (BMI). (See Box 3-4, "More muscle mass in older adults reduces the risk of dying prematurely.") In other words, exercise regularly and you might live longer.

Muscle mass loss

Low muscle mass is called sarcopenia and affects as many as 50 percent of older adults. Sarcopenia typically accelerates around age 75, although it may happen in people age 65 or 80. While it is a natural part of the aging process, your activity level often can dictate the speed at which you lose muscle mass (see Box 3-5, "Sarcopenia").

For instance, people who are physically inactive can lose as much as 3 to 5 percent of their muscle mass per decade after age 30. Low muscle mass means loss of strength and mobility, and can increase your risk of injuries from falls and contribute to weight gain.

Still, there are ways to slow the rate of sarcopenia. A review of more than 130 studies published in *Osteoporosis International* (December 2012) presented compelling evidence that specific dietary measures are needed in addition to resistance exercises to prevent the loss of muscle mass, strength, and performance in older adults. A group of 14 physicians and scientists reached the following conclusions:

 The intake of protein is an important component of muscle health. The recommended intake is 1.0–1.2 grams per 2.2 pounds of body weight per day. A study published in the

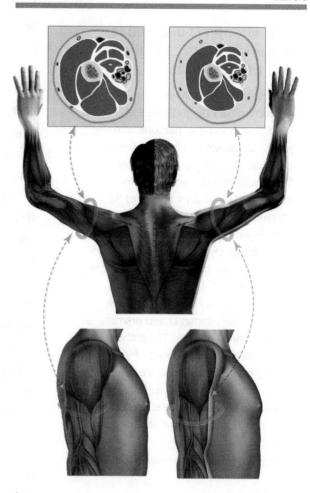

As you age, you lose lean muscle mass (left), which can result in a higher proportion of fat mass (right).

Low vitamin D in blood is associated with a higher risk of premature death

Scientists at the University of California, San Diego School of Medicine found that persons with low blood levels of vitamin D were twice as likely to die prematurely as those with higher levels. The findings were based on a review of 32 studies involving more than 566,000 people with an average age of 55 when the study began. Previous studies had shown that low vitamin D was associated with bone disease, but the current study establishes a link between low vitamin D and premature death from all causes. The authors concluded that high doses of vitamin D may be recommended for some patients under medical supervision. They add that everyone should consult their doctors before changing their intake of vitamin D.

American Journal of Public Health, June 12, 2014

☑ EASY TIP

PROPER NUTRITION IS IMPORTANT

Incorporate good nutrition before, during and after you participate in an exercise program. The combination of exercise and good nutrition is more beneficial than either good habit alone.

British Journal of Nutrition estimated a range of 40-70 grams per day, depending on the weight of the person.

▶ Vitamin D appears to be critical in the preservation of muscle mass and function. The findings indicate that vitamin D intake through diet, exposure to sunlight, and supplements is necessary for older adults (see Box 3-6, "Low vitamin D in blood is associated with a higher risk of premature death").

▶ The American Academy of Dermatology does not recommend sunlight as a means of obtaining vitamin D because of the risk of skin cancer, premature skin aging, and a weakened immune system. The need for supplemental vitamin D is particularly important among older patients who are hospitalized. The recommended daily intake of vitamin D for adults up to age 70 is 600 international units (IU). For those age 71 and older, it is 800 IU.

▶ Excessive intake of acid-producing foods, such as meat and grains, when combined with a low intake of alkalizing foods (like fruits and vegetables), may have a negative effect on muscle and bone health. The acidity of proteins has to be balanced by enough fruits and vegetables so the diet retains its alkaline nature. Diets high in alkaline-containing fruits and vegetables are associated with the preservation of lean tissue mass in older adults.

▶ Decreases in vitamin B-12 and folic acid intake may impair muscle function because of their action on homocysteine, an amino acid in blood plasma. A physician may recommend added vitamin B-12 through diet, with supplements, or by prescription medication. The recommended daily intake of vitamin B-12 is 2.4 micrograms (mcg).

The nutrition factor

Good nutrition alone can't prevent injuries, but there are connections between eating and exercise. Some, like hydration and what to eat before, during, and after exercise, have relatively short-term effects but are effective ways to ensure you maximize your workout effort and reduce your risk of injuries and soreness, and speed up recovery.

Short-term: Dealing with the stress of exercise

Proper nutrition and hydration can prepare your body to deal with the stress placed on it during exercise, making some injuries and conditions (cramps, for example) less likely. What you eat and when you eat it also have an effect on how you feel during exercise. Here are some nutrition and hydration suggestions designed for serious exercisers. (For beginners and older adults who may not exercise at an intense level, the rules are more flexible and should be based on what types of foods each individual tolerates.)

Hydration*

- Drink approximately 2-3 cups of water during the 2–3 hours before a strenuous exercise session.
- Drink approximately ½–1 cup of water every 15–20 minutes during a workout, but adjust amounts according to your body, the weather, and the intensity of your exercise.
- Drink approximately 2–4 cups of water after your workout for every pound of weight lost during your workout (weigh yourself immediately afterwards).

[* Adapted from the American College of Sports Medicine]

What to eat and drink before exercise

- Whole-grain cereals, bread
- Juice
- Fat-free yogurt
- Pancakes, waffles
- Fruits (apple or banana)

[*Adapted from Healthy Lifestyle Fitness, Mayo Clinic]

What to eat and drink after strenuous exercise (fluids, carbohydrates, protein)*

- Whole-grain English muffins, bagels, crackers
- Low-fat chocolate milk
- Juice/water blend
- Energy bars, low-fat granola bars
- Yogurt, bananas, and other fresh fruit
- Peanut butter sandwich
- Pretzels, pasta

[* Adapted from American Heart Association]

What's next?

Now that you have all the information you need to begin and maintain a core fitness program, it's time for action. Chapter 4, "Easy Exercises," outlines the three exercise programs of this report—strength, flexibility, and balance—which are designed specifically to meet your core fitness needs.

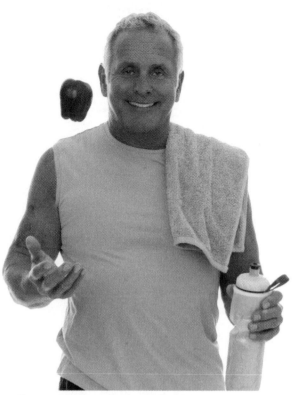

Proper nutrition and hydration before, during, and after exercise can fuel performance and reduce injuries.

☑ EASY TIP

KEEP HYDRATED
Don't wait until you are thirsty to drink fluids. Drink water before, during, and after exercise sessions.

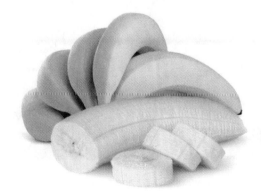

Fresh fruit, like bananas, offers a good amount of carbohydrates for pre-workout energy and post-exercise recovery.

4 EASY EXERCISES

Now that you have learned about your core, how it works, and why it's so important in maintaining optimal health, mobility, and wellness, it's time to learn the exercises that will help to strengthen and manage your core fitness.

The 50 exercises that make up *Easy Exercises for Core Fitness* are divided into three sections. Each one focuses on a specific area designed to improve your core. They include:

1. Strength
2. Flexibility
3. Balance

The directory

The directory highlighted on the opposite page lists the exercise number and what page they appear for easy reference. Each section is colored coded for better identification: blue for strength, green for flexibility, and yellow for balance.

The exercises

The illustrated instructions offer recommended number of reps and sets as well as variations for beginners and people with physical limitations. Many of the exercises use the equipment highlighted in Chapter 2, including stability and medicine balls, free weights, resistance bands, and even simple chairs, walls, and your own body weight. There is enough variety that you are bound to find many exercises that you enjoy and also are challenging, but can be performed safely and with comfort.

What's next?

In the next chapter, Chapter 5, "The Workbook," you will be shown how these exercises are placed into individual weekly programs for you to follow to ensure you get an all-around core fitness workout.

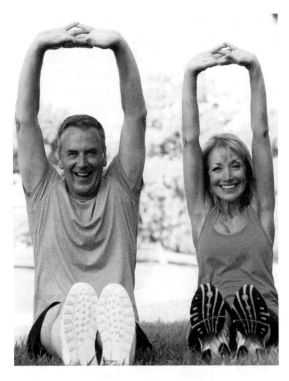

Right now is always the best time to adopt regular exercise. As you age, core fitness becomes crucial in maintaining a full and active lifestyle.

EASY EXERCISES DIRECTORY

Exercise Number   Page Number   Exercise Number   Page Number

CORE STRENGTH

1. Leg circles. 38
2. Superman 38
3. Plank. 38
4. Prone straight-leg raises. 39
5. Side leg lifts 39
6. Side plank. 39
7. Bracing 40
8. Bridges 40
9. Modified push-ups 40
10. Pendulum leg swings 41
11. Resistance band clamshells. 41
12. Resistance band squats 42
13. Resistance band standing row 42
14. Resistance band lat pull-downs 42
15. Shoulder squeeze. 43
16. Dumbbell curls 43
17. Dumbbell kneeling overhead press 43
18. Dumbbell overhead raises 43
19. Stability ball arm/leg extension. 44
20. Stability ball bridges 44
21. Stability ball push-ups 44
22. Medicine ball figure 8s 45
23. Wall push-ups. 45
24. Medicine ball cross-body swings 45

Strength programs 55

CORE FLEXIBILITY

25. Resistance band seated curls 46
26. Resistance band shoulder squeeze 46
27. Dead bug 46
28. Hip flexor stretches. 47
29. Lunges 47
30. Standing back extension 47
31. Side stretches. 47
32. Medicine ball overhead chops 48
33. Trunk curls 48
34. Sit backs. 48
35. Medicine ball twists 49
36. Stability ball arm/knee lifts 49
37. Stability ball hyperextension. 49
38. Reverse crunches. 50
39. Trunk lifts. 50
40. Hamstring stretches 50
41. Knees to chest 51
42. Pelvic tilt 51
43. Lumbar rotation 51
44. All-fours back extension. 51

Core programs 56

CORE BALANCE

45. Tandem walking 52
46. Single leg stand 52
47. Semi-sits. 52
48. Medicine ball overhead lunches 53
49. Stability ball wall squats 53
50. Stability ball bounce 53

Balance programs 57

LEG CIRCLES

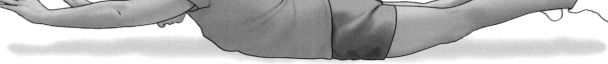

- ▶ Lie face-up on the floor or mat, legs extended comfortably, and tighten your stomach muscles.
- ▶ Lift your left leg 8-10 inches off the floor, move it in counterclockwise circles 8-10 times, then stop and reverse direction for another 8-10 circles.
- ▶ Stop, rest, then lift your right leg up and move it in counterclockwise circles 8-10 times, then stop and reverse direction for another 8-10 circles.
- ▶ Keep your abdominal muscles tight while performing leg circles, but don't hold your breath.

Variation for beginners and older adults: Complete 4-5 circles in both directions for both legs. This exercise may also be performed from a seated position.

SUPERMAN

- ▶ Lie face down on a floor or mat, arms extended forward.
- ▶ Tighten buttocks and lift your legs, shoulders, and arms off the floor simultaneously.
- ▶ Hold for 2-3 seconds and slowly return to the starting position.
- ▶ Work up to 8-10 repetitions, 2-3 sets.

Variation for beginners or older adults: Instead of lifting both arms and legs at the same time, lift your right arm and left leg. Complete as many reps as you can comfortably, then reverse the order and lift your left arm and right leg simultaneously.

PLANK

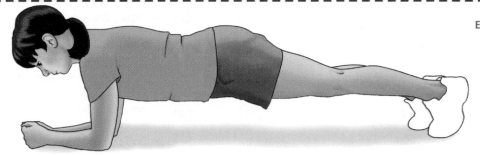

- ▶ Take a position on the floor or mat resting on your elbows and toes, head and neck in line with your body.
- ▶ Tighten your abs and position your body so it forms a straight line.
- ▶ Work up to holding that position for 5-10 seconds.
- ▶ Rest and complete 2-3 sets.

Variation for beginners and older adults: Hold the straight-line position for 3-5 seconds or as long as you can. Or hold the position on your knees instead of your toes.

PRONE STRAIGHT-LEG RAISES

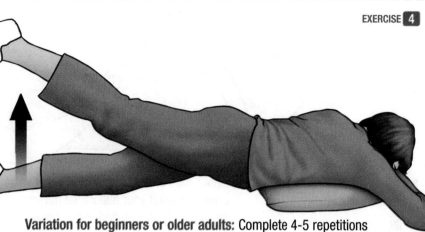

- Lie on your stomach with your abdomen, chest, and head supported with a cushion.
- Lock the right knee and raise the right leg at the hip. Avoid arching your back.
- Repeat the movement with the left leg.
- Work up to 8-10 repetitions for each leg, 2-3 sets (rest between sets).

Variation for beginners or older adults: Complete 4-5 repetitions and reduce the number of sets to 1-2 until you begin to increase strength.

SIDE LEG LIFTS

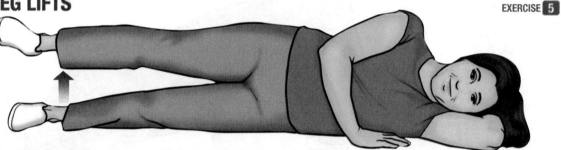

- Lie on your left side, right leg extended and on top of your left leg.
- Place your head on your left arm or on a cushion and place your right hand on the floor in front of you for balance.

- Slowly lift your right leg 12-18 inches and hold for 2-3 seconds.
- Slowly return to the starting position.
- Work up 8-10 repetitions and 2-3 sets.
- Change positions and perform the same exercise for the left leg.

Variation for beginners or older adults: Instead of lifting your entire leg, engage your abdominal muscles, squeeze your buttocks, and lift only your knee while keeping your heels together.

SIDE PLANK

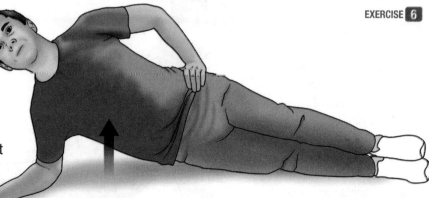

- Lie on your right side, right forearm supporting your upper body and the right side of the hips and legs touching the floor.
- Left hand on left hip.
- Contract your core muscles and lift your hips off the ground until your body is in a straight line.
- Hold for 2-3 seconds, relax, return to the starting position.
- Work up to 5 repetitions, 2-3 sets.

Variation for beginners and older adults: Lift your hips just off the floor instead of trying to form a straight line, and gradually work up to the straight-line position.

EASY EXERCISES FOR CORE STRENGTH

BRACING

EXERCISE **7**

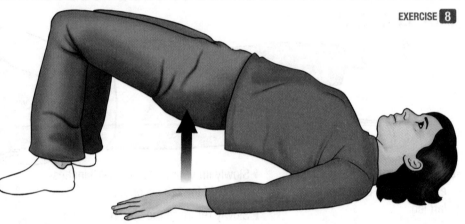

- Lie on your back, knees bent, feet flat on floor.
- Place your hands on your pelvis.

- Inhale, then exhale, and at the end of your exhale contract your abdominal muscles (think of getting punched in the stomach).
- Relax and work up to 8-10 times, 2-3 sets.

Variation for beginners and older adults: No variation needed, but lying on a relatively firm surface other than the floor also works.

BRIDGES

EXERCISE **8**

- Lie on your back, feet flat on the floor, arms extended at your sides.
- Contract your abdominal muscles and buttocks, and slowly raise your buttocks off the floor and up toward the ceiling. Do not arch your spine.
- Hold for 2-3 seconds and work up to 8-10 repetitions and 2-3 sets.

Variation for beginners and older adults: Restrict the upward movement of your hips/ buttocks and/or reduce the number of reps and sets.

MODIFIED PUSH-UPS

EXERCISE **9**

- Lie on your stomach, palms near your shoulders.
- Slowly move your head, neck, shoulders, and upper core upward, keeping your head up, and looking ahead.
- Lift upward until your arms are fully extended. Avoid arching your neck.
- Work up to 8-10 repetitions, 2-3 sets.

Variation for beginners and older adults: Restrict the distance your torso moves upward by not fully extending your arms.

PENDULUM LEG SWINGS

▶ Lie face-up on the floor or mat, tighten your abdominal muscles, and lift both legs upward as far as possible.

▶ Move both legs together from one side to the other, without touching the floor. This completes one repetition.

▶ Work up to 8-10 repetitions, 1 set only.

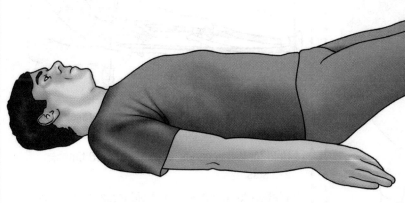

Variation for beginners and older adults: Keep knees bent and move both knees together from side to side, without touching the floor. Reduce the number of repetitions to 4-5.

RESISTANCE BAND CLAMSHELLS

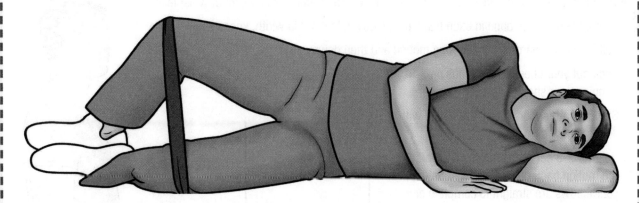

▶ Lie on your left side, right leg on top of the left, knees comfortably bent.

▶ With a resistance band wrapped around your knees, rotate the right leg up until your leg makes a 90-degree angle to the floor.

▶ Hold for 1-2 seconds and slowly return to the starting position.

▶ Work up to 8-10 repetitions, 2-3 sets.

▶ Change positions and complete the same number of repetitions and sets with the opposite leg.

Variation for beginners and older adults: Work up to 4-5 repetitions and 1-2 sets.

RESISTANCE BAND SQUATS EXERCISE 12

- Stand on a resistance band, legs at hip width.

- Hold one end of the band in each hand just below shoulder height.

- Slowly lower your body into a semi-sitting position, as if sitting in a chair, against the resistance of the band.

- Work up to 8-10 repetitions, 2-3 sets.

Variation for beginners and older adults: Lessen the tension of the band, complete 4-5 repetitions, and/or complete 1-2 sets.

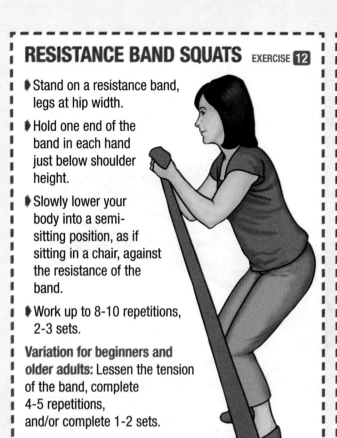

RESISTANCE BAND STANDING ROW EXERCISE 13

- Tie the middle of a resistance band around a doorknob or other fixed object at waist level.

- Hold one end of the band in each hand, feet at hip width, knees slightly bent.

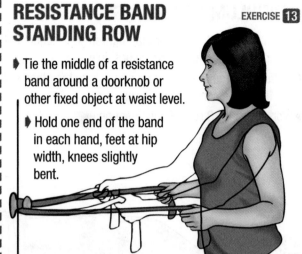

- Tighten your abs and pull the band parallel to the floor toward your body and to each side.

- Hold for 2-3 seconds, work up to 8-10 times, 2-3 sets.

Variation for beginners and older adults: Pull one side of the band at a time, and alternate sides; limit the hold phase to a count of one, reduce the number of repetitions to 4-5 and the number of sets to 1-2.

RESISTANCE BAND LAT PULL-DOWNS EXERCISE 14

- Tie the middle of a resistance band around a doorknob or other fixed object at waist level.

- Hold one end of the band in each hand, palms down, feet at hip width, knees slightly bent.

- Pull handles toward you in a rowing motion and then downwards.

- Stick out your chest as you focus on bringing your shoulder blades together.

- Stop just after your elbows are in line with your shoulders.

- Hold for 2-3 seconds and slowly reverse the motion back up and stop just before your elbows are straight to complete one repetition.

- Work up to 8-10 times, 2-3 sets.

Variation for beginners and older adults: Pull one side of the band at a time, and alternate sides; limit the hold phase to a count of one, reduce the number of repetitions to 4-5 and the number of sets to 1-2.

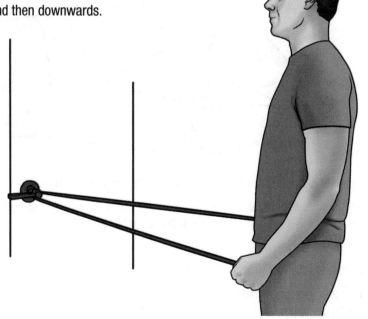

SHOULDER SQUEEZE

EXERCISE 15

- Stand straight, chest lifted, shoulders back and slightly down (not tensed).
- Arms to side, palms inward.
- Tighten your stomach muscles, squeeze your shoulder blades together, and hold for 5-10 seconds.
- Work up to 8-10 repetitions, 2-3 sets.

Variation for beginners or older adults: Hold for maximum of 5 seconds, 4-5 repetitions, 1-2 sets. This exercise may also be performed from a seated position.

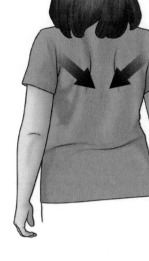

DUMBBELL CURLS

EXERCISE 16

- Hold a 1-5 pound dumbbell in each hand, arms down, palms out, and feet comfortably spread.
- Contract your abdominal muscles and move the weights upward by bending your elbows.
- Slowly lower the weights, stop, and repeat the movement.
- Work up to 8-10 repetitions, 2-3 sets.

Variation for beginners and older adults: Perform the lift alternately instead of simultaneously, lift a lighter weight, or reduce the number of repetitions to 4-5 and the number of sets to 1-2 until you begin to get stronger. This exercise also may be performed from a seated position.

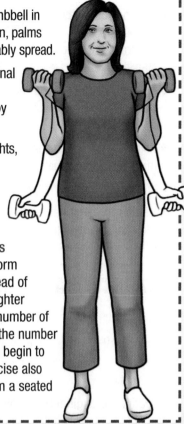

DUMBBELL KNEELING OVERHEAD PRESS

EXERCISE 17

- Bend your left knee and kneel on your right knee, left hand on hip.
- Hold a 1-2 pound dumbbell in your right hand at shoulder height.
- Raise the dumbbell by straightening (but not locking) your arm toward the ceiling. Switch leg/arm positions and repeat on the other side.
- Work up to 8-10 repetitions, 2-3 sets for each arm.

Variation for beginners and older adults: Start with 4-5 repetitions, 1-2 sets.

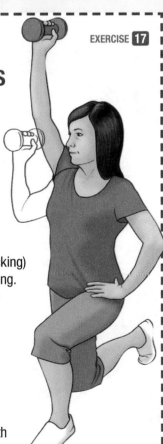

DUMBBELL OVERHEAD RAISES

EXERCISE 18

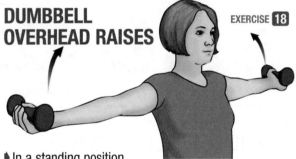

- In a standing position, hold a 1-5 pound dumbbell in each hand, elbows slightly bent, weights at shoulder height.
- Tighten your abdominal muscles and slowly lift both weights toward the ceiling without locking your elbows.
- Hold for 1-2 seconds, then slowly return to the starting position.
- Work up to 8-10 repetitions, 2-3 sets.

Variation for beginners and older adults: Perform the exercise sitting in a chair, lift lighter dumbbells, work up to 4-5 repetitions, and 1-2 sets until you get stronger.

STABILITY BALL ARM/LEG EXTENSION

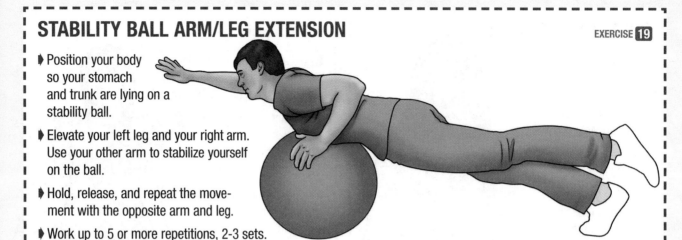

▶ Position your body so your stomach and trunk are lying on a stability ball.

▶ Elevate your left leg and your right arm. Use your other arm to stabilize yourself on the ball.

▶ Hold, release, and repeat the movement with the opposite arm and leg.

▶ Work up to 5 or more repetitions, 2-3 sets.

Variation for beginners and older adults: This is a difficult exercise, regardless of fitness level. If the stability ball makes the exercise too difficult, try doing it on the floor without the ball.

STABILITY BALL BRIDGES

▶ Lie face-up on the floor, stomach in (tight), shoulders flat, and place your feet on a stability ball, bench, or chair.

▶ Tighten your buttocks and raise your hips to create a straight line with your body.

▶ Hold for 2-3 seconds and then lower to the floor. Compete a set of 10 repetitions and work up to 2-3 sets.

Variation for beginners and older adults: Complete the same sequence of movements without the stability ball by lying on your back, feet flat on the floor. With stomach muscles tight, raise your hips and hold for 2-3 seconds. Complete 10 repetitions and work towards 2-3 sets.

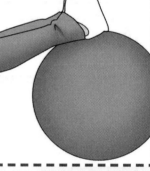

STABILITY BALL PUSH-UPS

▶ From a push-up position, extend your arms, place your hands on a stability ball, and pull in your stomach.

▶ Lower your chest as close as you can to the ball.

▶ Push back up, away from the ball.

▶ Repeat as many times as possible, using good form, and work up to a set of 10, then 2-3 sets of 10.

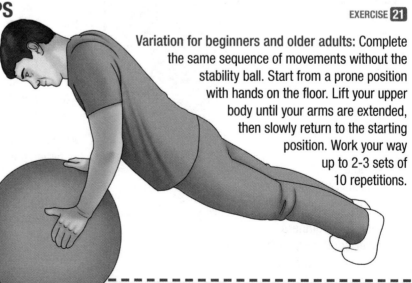

Variation for beginners and older adults: Complete the same sequence of movements without the stability ball. Start from a prone position with hands on the floor. Lift your upper body until your arms are extended, then slowly return to the starting position. Work your way up to 2-3 sets of 10 repetitions.

MEDICINE BALL FIGURE 8s EXERCISE 22

- From a standing position, feet at hip width, hold a medicine ball in front of your body, arms extended.

- Move the medicine ball in a side-to-side figure eight motion to complete 1 repetition.

- Work up to 8-10 repetitions, 2-3 sets.

Variation for beginners and older adults: Use a lighter medicine ball, complete 4-5 repetitions, or complete 1-2 sets. This exercise may be performed from a seated position.

WALL PUSH-UPS EXERCISE 23

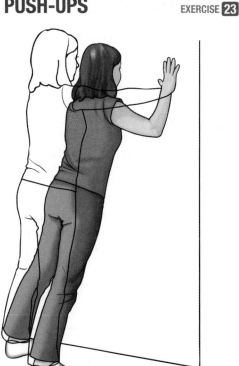

- Face a wall, arm's length away, feet at shoulder width.

- Lean forward, palms flat against the wall at shoulder height and shoulder-width apart.

- Bend your elbows and slowly lower your upper body toward the wall, keeping the feet flat.

- Hold for 1-2 seconds, then push back until your arms are straight.

- Repeat 8-12 times, rest, and complete one additional set of 8-12 reps.

MEDICINE BALL CROSS-BODY SWINGS EXERCISE 24

- Sit on the floor with knees bent and hold a medicine ball with both hands directly in front of and close to your body.

- Keep your trunk still and move your arms down and to the left side of your hip, then rotate them up, across your body, and above your right shoulder.

- Repeat the swing motion for up to 8-10 movements, then stop and reverse the motion (lower right to high left side), 2-3 sets.

Variation for beginners and older adults: Use a lighter ball or similar object, complete 4-5 repetitions on each side, or reduce the number of sets to 1-2. This exercise may be performed from a seated position by sitting toward the edge of the chair.

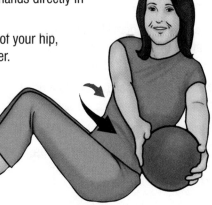

EASY EXERCISES FOR CORE STRENGTH

RESISTANCE BAND SEATED CURLS

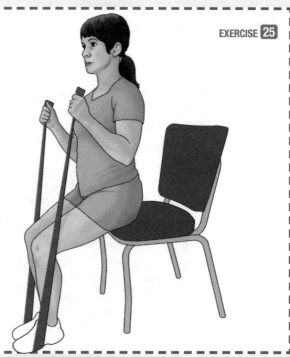

- Stand on a resistance band so that both feet anchor it to the floor.

- Hold the ends in both hands so that you feel a slight tension in the band.

- Tighten your stomach muscles and bend your elbow upward against the resistance of the band to a fully flexed position. Pause and then return to the starting position to complete 1 repetition.

- Work up to 8-10 repetitions, rest, and complete 2-3 more sets.

Variation for beginners and older adults: Reduce the number of repetitions to 4-5 and the number of sets to 1-2. Use a light free weight (1-5 pound dumbbell) to perform the curls instead of a resistance band.

RESISTANCE BAND SHOULDER SQUEEZE

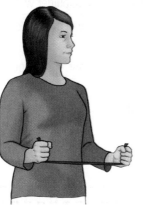 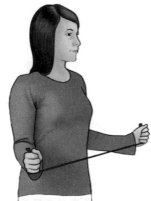

- Hold a resistance band in both hands, hands in front, elbows against sides and bent at a 90-degree angle.

- Squeeze your shoulders blades together as you rotate your arms away from your body, keeping elbows against sides.

- Hold for 2-3 seconds and return to the starting position.

- Work up to 8-10 repetitions, 2-3 sets.

Variation for beginners and older adults: Hold for a count of one, 4-5 repetitions, 1-2 sets.

DEAD BUG

- Lie on your back (no arch) and feet and knees off the floor and bent at 90 degrees.

- Tighten your abdominal muscles and extend your arms upward.

- Hold for 2-3 seconds, then slowly lower your right arm and left leg to the floor.

- Bring them back up, then lower your left arm and right leg to the floor to complete 1 repetition.

- Work up to 8-10 repetitions, 2-3 sets, but don't overdo it.

Variation for beginners and older adults: Begin with 4-5 repetitions. Hold for 1-2 seconds before lowering an arm or leg.

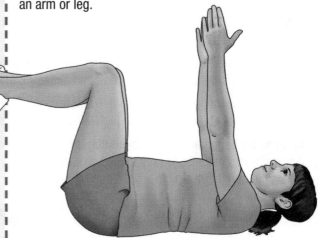

HIP FLEXOR STRETCHES

- Use a chair, counter, or wall for support and stand with your right leg forward, knee bent, left leg stretched behind you.
- Squeeze your buttocks and push forward with your pelvis.
- Hold for 20 seconds, relax, and repeat 2-3 times.
- Change position and perform the exercise with the left leg forward.

Variation for beginners and older adults: Hold for up to 10 seconds, then repeat the movement 1-2 times.

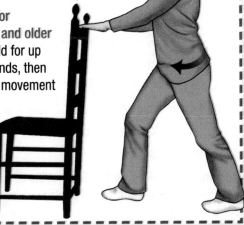

LUNGES

- Stand with your feet hip-width apart and then move your right foot forward 12-18 inches.
- Tighten your stomach muscles, slowly shift your weight forward, and bend the right knee.
- Keep the heel of the back foot on the floor.
- Slowly return to the starting position and relax. Switch legs and repeat the movement.
- Work up to 8-10 repetitions and 2-3 sets for each leg.
- Increase the load by holding 3-8 pound dumbbells in each hand.

Variation for beginners and older adults: Reduce the number of repetitions to 4-5 and the number of sets to 1-2 until you begin to get stronger.

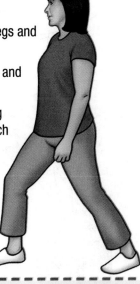

STANDING BACK EXTENSION

- Stand with feet slightly apart with hands on the small of your back.
- Slowly bend backward at the waist as far back as comfortable. Be careful not to overextend your neck.
- Slowly return to a neutral position.
- Work up to 8-10 repetitions, 2-3 sets

Variation for beginners and older adults: This is an easy exercise. No variation is needed other than reducing the number of repetitions and/or sets.

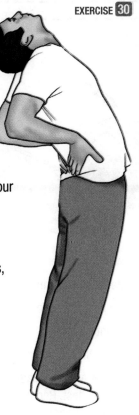

SIDE STRETCHES

- Lie on your back, legs straight.
- Bend your right leg and hold your knee or thigh with your left hand.
- Bring your bent leg across your body and toward the floor on your left side, while extending your right arm out to the side.
- Slowly return to the starting position and work up to 4-6 reps, 2-3 sets.
- Reverse leg positions and complete the same routine with your left leg and opposite hand/arm.

Variation for beginners and older adults: Reduce the number of repetitions to 2-4 and limit the number of sets to 1-2 until you are used to the exercise.

MEDICINE BALL OVERHEAD CHOPS

EXERCISE 32

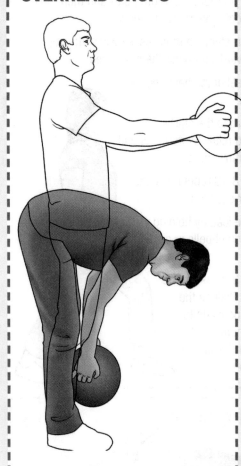

- Begin in a standing position, feet at hip-width distance, holding a medicine ball in front of your body.
- With abs engaged and straight back, bend at your hips and move the medicine ball forward, down, and between your legs in a chopping motion.
- Return to a straight-up position and swing the ball up and over your head to complete 1 repetition.
- Work up to 8-10 repetitions, 2-3 sets.

Variation for beginners and older adults: Use a lighter medicine ball, bring the ball back up only as high as your chest, or begin with 4-5 repetitions and/or 1-2 sets.

TRUNK CURLS

EXERCISE 33

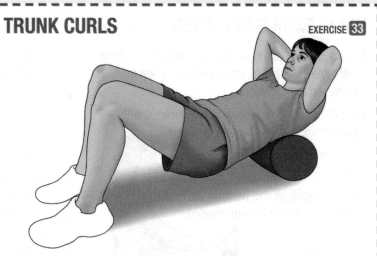

- Lie on your back with a foam roller positioned just below your shoulder blades.
- Knees bent, feet flat on the floor, hands behind head for support.
- Slowly raise your shoulders 6 inches.
- Hold for 2-3 seconds and slowly return to the starting position.
- Work up to 5 repetitions, 2-3 sets.

Variation for beginners and older adults: Restrict the upward movement to less than 6 inches, This exercise also can be done on the floor without a foam roller.

SIT BACKS

EXERCISE 34

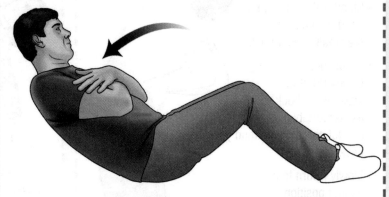

- Sit on the floor with knees bent and arms crossed across the chest.
- Tighten abdominal and back muscles.
- Lower upper body backwards for three counts, halfway to the floor
- Return to the upright position.
- Work up to 8-10 repetitions, 2-3 sets.

Variation for beginners and older adults: Sit at the edge of a chair, arms folded across the chest. Reduce the number of repetitions to 4-5 and/or reduce the number of sets to 1-2.

EASY EXERCISES FOR CORE FLEXIBILITY

MEDICINE BALL TWISTS

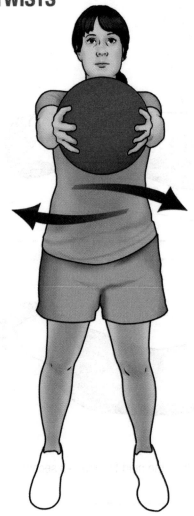

- Standing with feet hip-width apart, hold a medicine ball in front of your body, arms slightly bent.

- With stomach muscles contracted, swing the ball alternately to your right side and over your right hip, then across your body to the left side and over your left hip to complete 1 repetition.

- Work up to 8-10 repetitions, 2-3 sets.

Variation for beginners and older adults: Reduce the speed of ball movement as you swing your arms, reduce repetitions to 4-5, or limit sets to 1-2. This exercise also may be performed from a seated position.

STABILITY BALL ARM/KNEE LIFTS

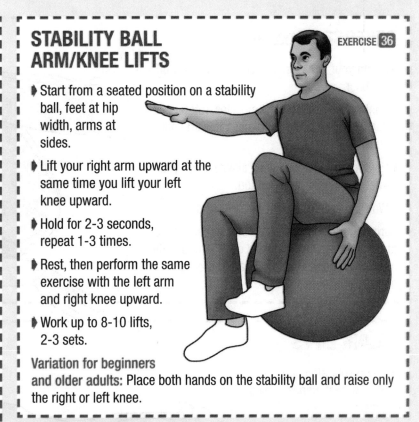

- Start from a seated position on a stability ball, feet at hip width, arms at sides.

- Lift your right arm upward at the same time you lift your left knee upward.

- Hold for 2-3 seconds, repeat 1-3 times.

- Rest, then perform the same exercise with the left arm and right knee upward.

- Work up to 8-10 lifts, 2-3 sets.

Variation for beginners and older adults: Place both hands on the stability ball and raise only the right or left knee.

STABILITY BALL HYPEREXTENSION

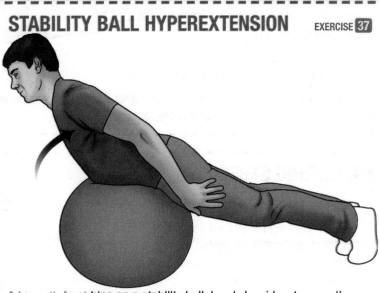

- Lie with front hips on a stability ball, hands by sides, toes on the floor.

- Tighten your buttocks, keep your lower body stable and lift your chest and shoulders.

- Hold for 2-3 seconds and return to the starting position.

- Work up to 8-10 repetitions and 2-3 sets.

Variation for beginners and older adults: Limit the distance of moving your shoulders and chest away from the ball and/or hold for 1-2 seconds instead of 2-3 seconds.

EASY EXERCISES FOR CORE FLEXIBILITY

REVERSE CRUNCHES

EXERCISE 38

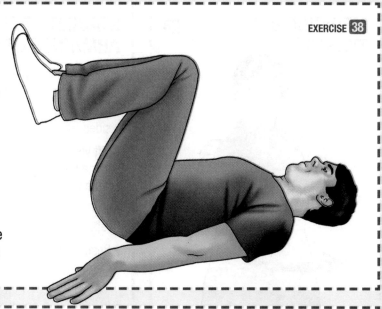

- Lie on your back, knees bent, feet slightly off the floor.
- Contract your abdominal muscles, rotate your pelvis up, and bring your knees toward your chest.
- Hold for 2-3 seconds, then slowly lower your knees to the starting position.
- Work up to 8-10 repetitions, 2-3 sets

Variation for beginners and older adults: Hold at the top for 1 count instead of 2-3, reduce the number of repetitions to 4-5, and/or reduce the number of sets to 1-2.

TRUNK LIFTS

EXERCISE 39

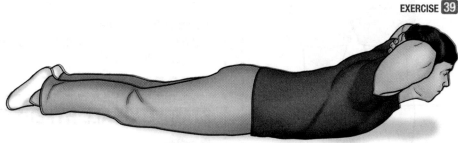

- Lie on your stomach, elbows bent, hands behind head.
- Without arching your neck, slowly lift your head and shoulders off the floor.
- Hold for 5 seconds and then lower down. Relax and repeat 5 times, 2-3 sets.

Variation for beginners and older adults: Restrict the upward motion and/or reduce the hold time to 2-3 seconds; perform 1-2 sets until you get used to the routine.

HAMSTRING STRETCHES

EXERCISE 40

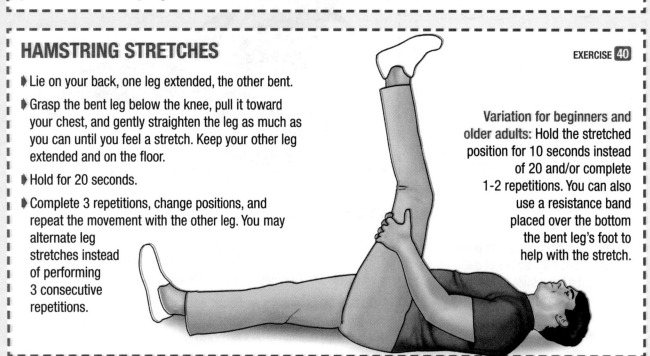

- Lie on your back, one leg extended, the other bent.
- Grasp the bent leg below the knee, pull it toward your chest, and gently straighten the leg as much as you can until you feel a stretch. Keep your other leg extended and on the floor.
- Hold for 20 seconds.
- Complete 3 repetitions, change positions, and repeat the movement with the other leg. You may alternate leg stretches instead of performing 3 consecutive repetitions.

Variation for beginners and older adults: Hold the stretched position for 10 seconds instead of 20 and/or complete 1-2 repetitions. You can also use a resistance band placed over the bottom the bent leg's foot to help with the stretch.

KNEES TO CHEST

- Lie on your back, knees bent slightly apart, and brought toward your body.
- Grasp behind your knees with both hands and pull them toward your chest.
- Hold for 10-20 seconds, return to the starting position, and repeat 2-3 times.

Variation for beginners and older adults: Pull one knee to your chest at a time, and/or reduce the number of repetitions to 1-2. This exercise also may be performed from a seated position.

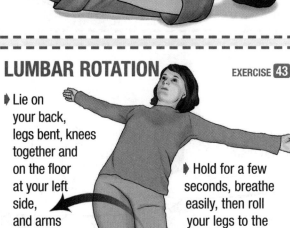

PELVIC TILT

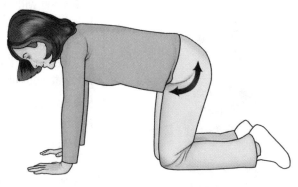

- From a starting position with hands and knees on the floor, pull in your stomach.
- Gently tilt your pelvis forward and backward 8-10 times while keeping your abs engaged and upper back stable.
- Rest, then complete another set of 8-10 reps.

Variation for beginners and older adults: Lie on your back with knees bent. Tighten your abdomen, squeeze your buttocks, and slightly rotate your pelvis up and off the floor. Hold for 2-3 seconds then rest. Reduce the number of repetitions to 4-5 or 1 set.

LUMBAR ROTATION

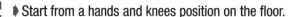

- Lie on your back, legs bent, knees together and on the floor at your left side, and arms extended outward. Try to keep your shoulders grounded.
- Engage your abs (in and up), keep your upper body still, and slowly roll your knees from the left to the right until they touch the floor, or come as close to the floor as possible without lifting your shoulders.

- Hold for a few seconds, breathe easily, then roll your legs to the opposite side to complete one repetition.
- Repeat 2-4 times to each side. Rest and complete 2-3 sets.

Variation for beginners and older adults: Reduce the number of reps to each side and/or the number of sets. Take 3-4 deep breaths after each rep.

ALL-FOURS BACK EXTENSION

- Start from a hands and knees position on the floor.
- Slowly lift and extend your left arm and right leg, hold for 2-3 seconds, then return to the starting position.
- Then slowly extend your right arm and left leg, holding for 2-3 seconds, to complete 1 repetition.
- Work up to 8-10 repetitions, 2-3 sets.

Variation for beginners and older adults: Just lift, rather than extend, your arms and legs. Reduce the number of reps and sets.

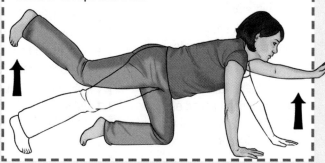

TANDEM WALKING

EXERCISE 45

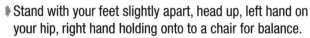

- Stand at one side of a long room.
- Contract your abs and place one foot in front of the other so that the heel of the forward foot touches the toes of the rear foot.
- Take 20 steps as if walking a tightrope.
- Turn and take 20 steps back to the starting point.
- Repeat 2-3 times, rest, and complete 2-3 sets.

Variation for beginners and older adults: Take 10 steps in each direction instead of 20, or complete 1-2 sets until you are comfortable doing the exercise.

SINGLE LEG STAND

EXERCISE 46

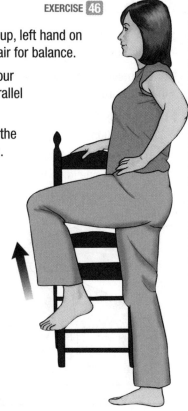

- Stand with your feet slightly apart, head up, left hand on your hip, right hand holding onto to a chair for balance.
- Tighten your stomach muscles and lift your left leg off the floor until your knee is parallel with your hip.
- Hold for 5 seconds, and slowly return to the starting position to complete 1 repetition.
- Work up to 8-10 repetitions and 2-3 sets.
- Change positions and repeat movement with the right leg.
- Gradually try to stand on the leg without holding onto the chair.

Variation for beginners and older adults: Limit the time balancing to 2-3 seconds, or complete 4-5 repetitions, 1-2 sets.

SEMI-SITS

EXERCISE 47

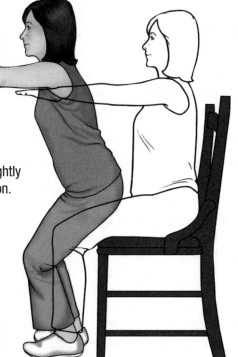

- Stand in front of a chair, feet hip-width apart.
- Engage your abdominal muscles by gently pulling them in and up.
- Slowly lower your buttocks and bend your knees as though you are going to sit.
- Instead, touch the chair seat lightly and return to a standing position.
- Work up to 8-10 repetitions, 2-3 sets.

Variation for beginners and older adults: Lower your buttocks just a few inches instead of going far enough to touch the chair seat. Restrict the number of repetitions to 4-5 and the number of sets to 1-2.

MEDICINE BALL OVERHEAD LUNGES

EXERCISE 48

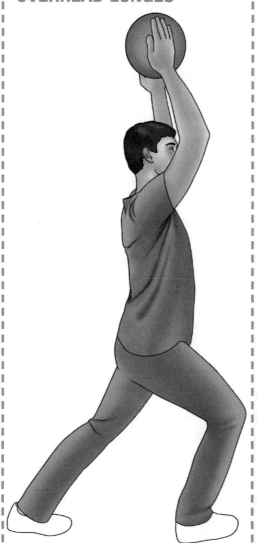

- Begin with feet together, holding a medicine ball over your head.

- Keep your abs tight and take one giant step forward with your right foot, keeping the medicine ball elevated, and lower your hips downward, weight on the forward foot.

- Slowly return to the starting position, then step forward with the left foot and return to starting position to complete 1 repetition.

- Work up to 8-10 repetitions, 2-3 sets.

Variation for beginners and older adults: Use a lighter medicine ball, complete 4-5 repetitions, or 1-2 sets.

STABILITY BALL WALL SQUATS

EXERCISE 49

- From a standing position, place the stability ball behind your back against a wall at waist level, hands to your sides.

- Slowly bend your knees into a semi-squat position, upper legs not quite parallel to the floor, allowing the ball to roll up your back.

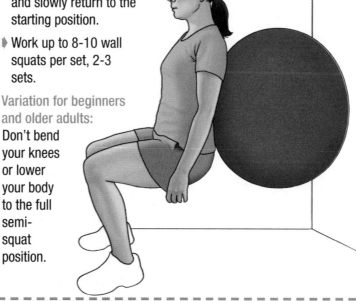

- Hold for 2-3 seconds, straighten your legs and slowly return to the starting position.

- Work up to 8-10 wall squats per set, 2-3 sets.

Variation for beginners and older adults: Don't bend your knees or lower your body to the full semi-squat position.

STABILITY BALL BOUNCE

EXERCISE 50

- Sit on a stability ball, feet spread, stomach in, and hands on hips.

- Gently bounce up and down while holding in your stomach muscles, using a spotter for safety.

- Bounce up to 8 or 10 times.

- Rest, and complete 2-3 sets.

Variation for beginners and older adults: Perform the stability ball bounce with arms and hands touching the ball for safety.

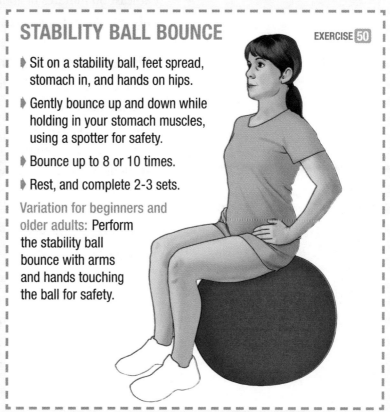

5 THE WORKBOOK

Now it is time to utilize the 50 exercises described here to improve your core fitness. Follow these guidelines:

☑ **Know your colors:** Each section—strength (blue), flexibility (green), and balance (yellow)—has four sample programs that mix and match the various exercises in those sections to offer a well-rounded routine designed to work that part of your core fitness.

☑ **Warm up and cool down with walking:** Every program also includes a 5-minute warm up before and a 5-minute cool down after. Walking is one of the easiest means to get the muscles and blood moving and to calm the body after exercise (see Box 2-8, "Proper walking techniques" on page 24).

☑ **Weekly workouts:** The workout schedule is based on a three-days-a-week routine with at least one day off in between. For instance, Monday, Wednesday, and Friday. As you progress, you can add a fourth day, if desired. On the other days, engage in at least 30 minutes of another activity that supports your core fitness, like walking, yoga, tai chi, or Pilates.

☑ **Monthly workout program:** A four-week workout schedule is offered on pages 58-59. The first two weeks are filled out for you, and include a checklist to note when your workout is completed and a place to add personal comments. For the last two weeks, simply choose a program of your liking from the three color-coded sections, or create your own from the different exercises within that category.

☑ **Core fitness for sports:** Finally, if are involved in a sport or activity, there are all-around core-building routines to help you improve your performance and overall fitness in those endeavors.

Easy Exercises for Core Fitness can help you improve one of the most essential areas of your wellness. With a strong, flexible, and balanced core, you are able to stay healthy and enjoy a longer, active, and productive life.

EASY STRENGTH PROGRAM #1

☑ Warm up: 5 minutes

☑ **SUPERMAN OR STABILITY BALL ARM/LEG EXTENSION**
- Exercise: **2 or 19**
- Reps: 8-10
- Sets: 2-3

☑ **PLANK**
- Exercise: **3**
- Hold position: 5-10 seconds
- Sets: 2-3

☑ **MODIFIED PUSH-UPS**
- Exercise: **9**
- Reps: 8-10
- Sets: 2-3

☑ **SIDE LEG LIFTS**
- Exercise: **5**
- Reps: 8-10
- Sets: 2-3

☑ Cool down: 5 minutes

EASY STRENGTH PROGRAM #2

☑ Warm up: 5 minutes

☑ **SUPERMAN OR PRONE STRAIGHT-LEG RAISES**
- Exercise: **2 or 4**
- Reps: 8-10
- Sets: 2-3

☑ **PLANK OR SIDE PLANK**
- Exercise: **3 or 6**
- Plank hold position: 5-10 seconds
- Side plank hold position: 2-3 seconds
- Sets: 2-3

☑ **STABILITY BALL PUSH-UPS**
- Exercise: **21**
- Reps: 8-10
- Sets: 1-2

☑ **SIDE LEG LIFTS OR RESISTANCE BAND CLAMSHELLS**
- Exercise: **5 or 11**
- Reps: 8-10
- Sets: 2-3

☑ Cool down: 5 minutes

EASY STRENGTH PROGRAM #3

☑ Warm up: 5 minutes

☑ **BRIDGES OR STABILITY BALL BRIDGES**
- Exercise: **8 or 20**
- Reps: 8-10
- Sets: 2-3

☑ **LEG CIRCLES**
- Exercise: **1**
- Reps: 8-10 circles in each direction
- Sets: 1-2 sets for each leg

☑ **RESISTANCE BAND STANDING ROW**
- Exercise: **13**
- Reps: 8-10
- Sets: 2-3

☑ **WALL PUSH-UPS**
- Exercise: **23**
- Reps: 8-10
- Sets: 2-3

☑ Cool down: 5 minutes

EASY STRENGTH PROGRAM #4

☑ Warm up: 5 minutes

☑ **PENDULUM LEG SWINGS**
- Exercise: **10**
- Reps: 8-10
- Sets: 1

☑ **BRACING**
- Exercise: **7**
- Reps: 8-10 circles in each direction
- Sets: 1, 2, or 3 for each leg

☑ **DUMBBELL OVERHEAD RAISES**
- Exercise: **18**
- Reps: 8-10
- Sets: 2-3

☑ **SHOULDER SQUEEZE OR WALL PUSH-UPS**
- Exercise: **15 or 23**
- Reps: 8-10
- Sets: 2-3

☑ Cool down: 5 minutes

EASY FLEXIBILITY PROGRAM #1

☑ Warm up: 5 minutes

☑ **DEAD BUG**
- Exercise: 27
- Reps: 8-10
- Sets: 2-3

☑ **LUMBAR ROTATION**
- Exercise: 43
- Reps: 2-4
- Sets: 2-3

☑ **LUNGES**
- Exercise: 29
- Reps: 8-10
- Sets: 2-3

☑ **STANDING BACK EXTENSION**
- Exercise: 30
- Reps: 8-10
- Sets: 2-3

☑ Cool down: 5 minutes

EASY FLEXIBILITY PROGRAM #2

☑ Warm up: 5 minutes

☑ **KNEES TO CHEST**
- Exercise: 41
- Hold position: 10-20 seconds
- Sets: 2-3

☑ **SIDE STRETCHES**
- Exercise: 31
- Reps: 8-10
- Sets: 2-3

☑ **TRUNK CURLS OR TRUNK LIFTS**
- Exercise: 33 or 39
- Reps: 5
- Sets: 2-3

☑ **PELVIC TILT**
- Exercise: 42
- Reps: 8-10
- Sets: 1-2

☑ Cool down: 5 minutes

EASY FLEXIBILITY PROGRAM #3

☑ Warm up: 5 minutes

☑ **REVERSE CRUNCHES**
- Exercise: 38
- Reps: 8-10
- Sets: 2-3

☑ **STABILITY BALL ARM/KNEE LIFTS**
- Exercise: 36
- Reps: 8-10
- Sets: 2-3

☑ **SIT BACKS**
- Exercise: 34
- Reps: 8-10
- Sets: 2-3

☑ **RESISTANCE BAND SEATED CURLS**
- Exercise: 25
- Reps: 8-10
- Sets: 2-3

☑ Cool down: 5 minutes

EASY FLEXIBILITY PROGRAM #4

☑ Warm up: 5 minutes

☑ **ALL-FOURS BACK EXTENSION**
- Exercise: 44
- Reps: 8-10
- Sets: 2-3

☑ **HAMSTRING STRETCHES**
- Exercise: 40
- Hold position: 20 seconds
- Sets: 2-3

☑ **HIP FLEXOR STRETCHES**
- Exercise: 28
- Hold position: 20 seconds
- Sets: 2-3

☑ **RESISTANCE BAND SHOULDER SQUEEZE**
- Exercise: 26
- Reps: 8-10
- Sets: 2-3

☑ Cool down: 5 minutes

EASY BALANCE PROGRAM #1

- ☑ Warm up: 5 minutes
- ☑ **TANDEM WALKING**
  - Exercise: 45
  - Reps: 2-3
  - Sets: 2-3
- ☑ **SINGLE LEG STAND**
  - Exercise: 46
  - Reps: 8-10
  - Sets: 2-3
- ☑ **SEMI-SITS**
  - Exercise: 47
  - Reps: 8-10
  - Sets: 2-3
- ☑ **DUMBBELL KNEELING OVERHEAD PRESS**
  - Exercise: 17
  - Reps: 8-10
  - Sets: 2-3 with each arm
- ☑ Cool down: 5 minutes

EASY BALANCE PROGRAM #2

- ☑ Warm up: 5 minutes
- ☑ **TANDEM WALKING**
  - Exercise: 45
  - Reps: 2-3
  - Sets: 2-3
- ☑ **STABILITY BALL WALL SQUATS**
  - Exercise: 49
  - Reps: 8-10
  - Sets: 2-3
- ☑ **STABILITY BALL BOUNCE**
  - Exercise: 50
  - Reps: 8-10
  - Sets: 2-3
- ☑ **STANDING BACK EXTENSION**
  - Exercise: 30
  - Reps: 8-10
  - Sets: 2-3
- ☑ Cool down: 5 minutes

EASY BALANCE PROGRAM #3

- ☑ Warm up: 5 minutes
- ☑ **MEDICINE BALL OVERHEAD CHOPS**
  - Exercise: 32
  - Reps: 8-10
  - Sets: 2-3
- ☑ **LUNGES OR MEDICINE BALL OVERHEAD LUNGES**
  - Exercise: 29 or 48
  - Reps: 8-10
  - Sets: 2-3
- ☑ **MEDICINE BALL TWISTS**
  - Exercise: 35
  - Reps: 8-10
  - Sets: 2-3
- ☑ **MEDICINE BALL FIGURE 8s**
  - Exercise: 22
  - Reps: 8-10
  - Sets: 2-3
- ☑ Cool down: 5 minutes

EASY BALANCE PROGRAM #4

- ☑ Warm up: 5 minutes
- ☑ **SINGLE-LEG STAND**
  - Exercise: 46
  - Reps: 8-10
  - Sets: 2-3
- ☑ **RESISTANCE BAND SQUATS**
  - Exercise: 12
  - Reps: 8-10
  - Sets: 2-3
- ☑ **DUMBBELL KNEELING OVERHEAD PRESS**
  - Exercise: 17
  - Reps: 8-10
  - Sets: 2-3
- ☑ **TANDEM WALKING OR SEMI-SITS**
  - Exercise: 45 or 47
  - Tandem walking reps: 2-3
  - Semi-sits reps: 8-10
  - Sets: 2-3
- ☑ Cool down: 5 minutes

WEEK #1

EXERCISE DAY OF THE WEEK	CORE STRENGTH PROGRAM (SEE PAGE 55)	CORE FLEXIBILITY PROGRAM (SEE PAGE 56)	CORE BALANCE PROGRAM (SEE PAGE 57)	☑ CHECK WHEN COMPLETED	COMMENTS
MONDAY	Program #1	✗	Program #1		
TUESDAY	☑ walking ☑ **yoga** ☑ tai chi ☑ pilates				
WEDNESDAY	Program #2	Program #1	✗		
THURSDAY	☑ **walking** ☑ yoga ☑ tai chi ☑ pilates				
FRIDAY	✗	Program #2	Program #2		
SATURDAY	☑ **walking** ☑ yoga ☑ tai chi ☑ pilates				
SUNDAY	OFF				

WEEK #2

EXERCISE DAY OF THE WEEK	CORE STRENGTH PROGRAM (SEE PAGE 55)	CORE FLEXIBILITY PROGRAM (SEE PAGE 56)	CORE BALANCE PROGRAM (SEE PAGE 57)	☑ CHECK WHEN COMPLETED	COMMENTS
MONDAY	Program #3	✗	Program #3		
TUESDAY	☑ walking ☑ **yoga** ☑ tai chi ☑ pilates				
WEDNESDAY	Program #4	Program #3	✗		
THURSDAY	☑ **walking** ☑ yoga ☑ tai chi ☑ pilates				
FRIDAY	✗	Program #4	Program #4		
SATURDAY	☑ **walking** ☑ yoga ☑ tai chi ☑ pilates				
SUNDAY	OFF				

EXERCISE DAY OF THE WEEK	CORE STRENGTH PROGRAM (SEE PAGE 55)	CORE FLEXIBILITY PROGRAM (SEE PAGE 56)	CORE BALANCE PROGRAM (SEE PAGE 57)	☑ CHECK WHEN COMPLETED	COMMENTS
MONDAY					
TUESDAY					
WEDNESDAY					
THURSDAY					
FRIDAY					
SATURDAY					
SUNDAY					

WEEK #3

EXERCISE DAY OF THE WEEK	CORE STRENGTH PROGRAM (SEE PAGE 55)	CORE FLEXIBILITY PROGRAM (SEE PAGE 56)	CORE BALANCE PROGRAM (SEE PAGE 57)	☑ CHECK WHEN COMPLETED	COMMENTS
MONDAY					
TUESDAY					
WEDNESDAY					
THURSDAY					
FRIDAY					
SATURDAY					
SUNDAY					

WEEK #4

EASY EXERCISE MONTHLY WORKBOOK

EASY EXERCISE ACTIVITY AND SPORTS PROGRAMS

THREE FOR
GOLF

☑ **Warm up:** 5 minutes

☑ **MEDICINE BALL CROSS-BODY SWINGS**
- Exercise: **24**
- Reps: 8-10
- Sets: 2-3

☑ **STABILITY BALL HYPEREXTENSION**
- Exercise: **37**
- Reps: 8-10
- Sets: 2-3

☑ **MEDICINE BALL TWISTS**
- Exercise: **35**
- Reps: 8-10
- Sets: 2-3

☑ **Cool down:** 5 minutes

THREE FOR
TENNIS

☑ **Warm up:** 5 minutes

☑ **MEDICINE BALL TWISTS**
- Exercise: **35**
- Reps: 8-10
- Sets: 2-3

☑ **MEDICINE BALL OVERHEAD CHOPS**
- Exercise: **32**
- Reps: 8-10
- Sets: 2-3

☑ **STABILITY BALL WALL SQUATS**
- Exercise: **49**
- Reps: 8-10
- Sets: 2-3

☑ **Cool down:** 5 minutes

THREE FOR
SWIMMING

☑ **Warm up:** 5 minutes

☑ **DUMBBELL OVERHEAD RAISES**
- Exercise: **18**
- Reps: 8-10
- Sets: 2-3

☑ **RESISTANCE BAND LAT PULL-DOWNS**
- Exercise: **14**
- Reps: 8-10
- Sets: 2-3

☑ **STABILITY BALL WALL SQUATS**
- Exercise: **49**
- Reps: 8-10
- Sets: 2-3

☑ **Cool down:** 5 minutes

THREE FOR
BICYCLING

☑ **Warm up:** 5 minutes

☑ **MEDICINE BALL CROSS-BODY SWINGS**
- Exercise: **24**
- Reps: 8-10
- Sets: 2-3

☑ **BRIDGES**
- Exercise: **8**
- Reps: 8-10
- Sets: 2-3

☑ **PELVIC TILTS**
- Exercise: **42**
- Reps: 8-10
- Sets: 2-3

☑ **Cool down:** 5 minutes

THREE FOR
BOWLING

- ☑ **Warm up:** 5 minutes

- ☑ **MEDICINE BALL CROSS-BODY SWINGS**
  - Exercise: **24**
  - Reps: 8-10
  - Sets: 2-3

- ☑ **KNEES TO CHEST**
  - Exercise: **41**
  - Reps: 2-3
  - Sets: 2-3

- ☑ **MEDICINE BALL TWISTS**
  - Exercise: **35**
  - Reps: 8-10
  - Sets: 2-3

- ☑ **Cool down:** 5 minutes

THREE FOR
HIKING

- ☑ **Warm up:** 5 minutes

- ☑ **SIDE LEG LIFTS**
  - Exercise: **5**
  - Reps: 8-10
  - Sets: 2-3

- ☑ **BRIDGES**
  - Exercise: **8**
  - Reps: 8-10
  - Sets: 2-3

- ☑ **PELVIC TILTS**
  - Exercise: **42**
  - Reps: 8-10
  - Sets: 2-3

- ☑ **Cool down:** 5 minutes

THREE FOR
RUNNING

- ☑ **Warm up:** 5 minutes

- ☑ **SIDE PLANK**
  - Exercise: **6**
  - Reps: 5
  - Sets: 2-3

- ☑ **BRIDGES**
  - Exercise: **8**
  - Reps: 8-10
  - Sets: 2-3

- ☑ **RESISTANCE BAND CLAMSHELLS**
  - Exercise: **11**
  - Reps: 8-10
  - Sets: 2-3

- ☑ **Cool down:** 5 minutes

THREE FOR
HOUSEWORK/ YARDWORK

- ☑ **Warm up:** 5 minutes

- ☑ **SHOULDER SQUEEZE**
  - Exercise: **15**
  - Reps: 8-10
  - Sets: 2-3

- ☑ **STANDING BACK EXTENSION**
  - Exercise: **30**
  - Reps: 8-10
  - Sets: 2-3

- ☑ **DUMBBELL CURLS**
  - Exercise: **16**
  - Reps: 8-10
  - Sets: 2-3

- ☑ **Cool down:** 5 minutes

EASY EXERCISE ACTIVITY AND SPORTS PROGRAMS

APPENDIX I: GLOSSARY

ABDOMINALS (ABS): the muscles that support the area of the body between the chest and the pelvis

AEROBIC EXERCISE: physical activity that increases the intake of oxygen and improves the cardiovascular and respiratory systems

BALANCE: the even distribution of weight that enables a person to remain upright and steady; also called equilibrium

BALLISTIC STRETCHING: a form of stretching that uses the momentum to force a muscle group or joint beyond its normal range of motion

BODY MASS INDEX: a formula for categorizing weight in relation to height

BODY WEIGHT EXERCISES: a type of exercise in which the weight of your body is used as resistance (example: modified push-ups)

CORE: the muscles of the hips, pelvis, trunk, shoulders, and neck

CRAMP: a sudden, involuntary, painful contraction of a muscle

EXTENSION: straightening or extending a joint or limb of the body

FLEXION: bending a joint or limb of the body

FLEXIBILITY: the range of motion through which a joint moves

FOAM ROLLER: a cylindrically shaped exercise device made of a foam product that is used as a form of self-massage or to loosen muscle tissue

FREE WEIGHTS: dumbbells, barbells, or kettlebells, for example, used in resistance training

HAMSTRING: a muscle or tendon behind the upper part of the legs

LIGAMENT: a tissue that connects bones or cartilages

MEDICINE BALL: a heavy, solid ball used in resistance training

MOBILITY: the ability to move in one's environment with ease and without restriction

MUSCLE IMBALANCE: refers to opposite muscle groups (biceps/triceps, for example) that are not balanced in terms of strength

MYOFASCIAL RELEASE: a type of therapy used to ease soft muscle tissue stiffness and pain

NEUTRAL SPINE POSITION: one in which there are natural curves of the cervical spine/neck, thoracic spine/mid back, and lumbar spine/lower back

OBESITY: a higher level of being overweight in relation to height, sometimes defined as being 20 percent more than healthy weight

OSTEOARTHRITIS (OA): a disease characterized by the degeneration of cartilage and the underlying bone

OSTEOPENIA: lower than normal bone density

OSTEOPOROSIS: a disease in which the bones become weak, brittle, and porous

OVERWEIGHT: a weight that is not healthy for a person of a given height

PILATES: an exercise program that consists of 25 to 50 low-impact strength and endurance movements that may improve posture, balance, and flexibility

QUADRICEPS: large muscles on the upper front area of the legs

REPETITION (REP): the single act of lifting or moving a part of the body against resistance

RESISTANCE BANDS: elastic bands that act as resistance against movement during resistance training

RESISTANCE TRAINING: a form of exercise that involves movement or attempted movement against resistance (or load); also called weight training

SARCOPENIA: age-related loss of muscle mass and strength

SET: the number of repetitions of an exercise movement

SPRAIN: an injury caused by forcing a joint beyond its normal range of motion

STABILITY BALL: a large, inflatable ball used in various exercises

STRAIN: a stretched or torn muscle or tendon, informally referred to as a pulled muscle

STRENGTH: the ability to exert force against resistance

SUPINATION: the action of the feet in which they roll outward when running or walking; also called under-pronation

TAI CHI: a combination of relaxation, meditation, deep breathing, and slow, gentle, continuous, and structured exercises

TENDON: a tissue that connects muscles to bones and cartilage

30-SECOND SIT-TO-STAND CHAIR TEST: used to measure core and leg strength and endurance.

TORSO: the trunk of the body

WEIGHT TRAINING: also called resistance training, in which a person lifts or moves weights in order to gain muscle strength or endurance

YOGA: a type of exercise that incorporates movement, relaxation, and gentle breathing that may lead to improved balance, flexibility, range of motion, and strength

APPENDIX II: RESOURCES

American Academy of Orthopaedic Surgeons
6300 N. River Road
Rosemont, IL 60018
847-823-7186
www.aaos.org

American Academy of Physical Medicine & Rehabilitation
9700 West Bryn Mawr Avenue, Suite 200
Rosemont, IL 600185701
847-737-6000
www.aapmr.org

American College of Sports Medicine
401 West Michigan Street
Indianapolis, IN 46202-3233
317-637-9200
www.acsm.org

American Council on Exercise
4851 Paramount Drive
San Diego, CA 92123
888-825-3636
www.acefitness.org

American Physical Therapy Association
1111 North Fairfax Street
Alexandria, VA 22314-1488
800-999-2782
www.apta.org/BalanceFalls

Arthritis Foundation
1330 W. Peachtree Street, Suite 100
Atlanta, GA 30309
404-872-7100
www.arthritis.org

Centers for Disease Control and Prevention
1600 Clifton Road
Atlanta, GA 30333
800-232-4636
www.cdc.gov

Center for Healthy Aging
c/o National Council on Aging
1901 L Street, NW, 4th Floor
Washington, D.C. 20036
202-479-1200
www.ncoa.org/improve-health/center-for-healthy-aging

David Geffen School of Medicine at UCLA
Division of Geriatrics
10945 Le Conte Avenue, Suite 2339
Los Angeles, CA 90095
800-825-2631

Department of Rehabilitation Services
UCLA Health System
757 Westwood Boulevard., Suite 3127
Los Angeles, CA 90094
310-825-5650
www.rehab.ucla.edu

Fall Prevention Center of Excellence
University of Southern California Andrus Gerontology Center
3715 McClintock Avenue., Room 228
Los Angeles, CA 90089-0191
213-740-1364
www.stopfalls.org

National Council on Aging
1901 L Street, NW, 4th Floor
Washington, DC 20036
202-479-1200
www.ncoa.org

National Institute on Aging
31 Center Drive, MSC 2292
Bethesda, MD 20892
800-222-2225
www.nia.nih.gov

National Safety Council
1121 Spring Lake Drive
Itasca, IL 60143-3201
800-621-7615
www.nsc.org

National Strength and Conditioning Association
1885 Bob Johnson Drive
Colorado Springs, CO 80906
719-632-6722
www.nsca.com

U.S. Department of Veterans Affairs
810 Vermont Avenue, NE
Washington, DC 20420
www.patientsafety.gov